THE IDEA OF HEALTH

Implications for the Nursing Professional

NURSING EDUCATION SERIES

DOROTHY SMITH and MARY RANSHORN, *Editors*

Judith A. Smith, *The Idea of Health: Implications
for the Nursing Professional*

THE IDEA OF HEALTH

Implications for the Nursing Professional

JUDITH A. SMITH, PH.D., R.N.
University of Pennsylvania

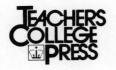

Teachers College, Columbia University
New York and London   1983

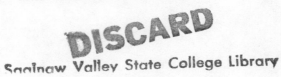

Published by Teachers College Press, 1234 Amsterdam Avenue, New York, N.Y. 10027

Library of Congress Cataloging in Publication Data

Smith, Judith A., 1941–
   The idea of health.

   (Nursing education series)
   Bibliography: p.
   Includes index.
   1. Nursing—Philosophy. 2. Health. I. Title.
II. Series. [DNLM: 1. Health—Nursing texts.
2. Philosophy, Nursing. WY 86 S653i]
RT 84.5.S57 1983   610.73'01   83-389

ISBN 0-8077-2735-0 (pbk.)

Manufactured in the United States of America

88 87 86 85 84 83   1 2 3 4 5 6

CONTENTS

PREFACE

There is a need for the clarification of the idea of health. Modern society has seen the rise of a variety of organizations and professions supplementary or parallel to the practice of the physician. The rise of health institutes, independent nursing practices, and community health agencies has created situations that implicitly demand a clarification of their objectives and relationships to the traditional aims of medicine. This book is an analysis of the aims and methods of the delivery of health care in modern society.

The book is divided into four general areas. One area focuses on the inevitable historical links between nurses and physicians and an analysis of the new horizons in nursing that anticipate practice as independent from, rather than subordinate to, the practice of the physician.

The second section presents an exposition and analysis of the idea of health characteristic of ancient Greek thought and its relationship to the rise of public health in modern times. The ancient Greek idea of health and health care was conceived as the focus of culture and education—in a word, as *paideia*. This classical view of health embraced the total human condition. It found expression in the Hippocratic treatises and was part of the general philosophical climate of the age of Plato and Aristotle.

The aim of this area is to survey and identify certain distinctive features of ancient Greek medicine and to show that certain comparable developments played a role in the rise of modern public health.

The third area is an exposition and analysis of four distinctive ideas of health. They are presented as four ways of conceiving the health-illness continuum and as four models of health care. These models were chosen because of their significance as directive ideas in the practice of the restoration and preservation of health and also because they play a significant role in the writings of a number of important contemporary researchers. The discussion of these four models is presented as a critical examination of the writings of representative authors. One outcome of the inquiry has been the recognition of the progressively inclusive character of these four concepts of health. It appears that what is here called the eudaimonistic model of health embraces the concerns of the other three and presents a model of health care very close to the comprehensive ideal of paideia in ancient Greek philosophy.

Since the motivation for this inquiry and my primary professional interest is nursing, a fourth section discusses the implications of this inquiry for the nursing profession. This discussion is presented in three parts. The first discusses the general structure and interrelationships of the models of health. The second indicates the direct impact of this inquiry on education, practice, and research in the nursing profession. The third considers the implications of these models for ethical ideals of man and society, the four models being viewed as related to four different conceptions of human life and levels of social action affecting the varied goals of nursing.

Chapter 9, General Structure and Interrelationships of the Four Models, is devoted to the discussion of the nursing profession as contrasted with the traditional role of the medical doctor. This subject has been receiving increasing attention and has led to a tendency to stress the independence of nursing from the physician. Nevertheless, we cannot overlook the fact that the practices of both nurse and physician are part of the larger social enterprise traditionally designated by the word medicine. In this book, the word "medicine" is used in this larger sense; it means the accumulated sciences, arts, and techniques of restoring and preserving health. Briefly then, medicine as used here means the cultivation of health. No other term is appropriate for this purpose.

The only place in this book that the word medicine is used in the narrower sense in which it refers only to the practice of the physician is in Chapter 5, Clinical Model, where its restricted meaning is quite clear.

From the viewpoint of the newly emerging professional independence of nursing, objections will be raised to the use of the term medicine. Granted, that in a sense nursing is not to be identified with medicine—but in that sense the physician's practice is not to be identified with medicine either. Both, however independent of each other, are undeniably part of the more general category that is designated by the term medicine. Objection to this usage is no more valid than objection to the general term European on the ground that a German is not a Frenchman.

I am indebted to Professor William Gruen, professor emeritus of New York University, for many of the ideas in this book are based on what was derived from his course in the Philosophy of Science.

—J.A.S.

Chapter 1

INTRODUCTION

Fundamental to any development of community health[1] policy and practice is the idea of health itself. What is the healthy person? The answer varies according to the perspective of the respondent.[2] For example, it could be couched in terms of physiology, with health being defined as the optimal functioning of organ systems. Or it could be conceived economically, health being regarded as the condition in which economic man fulfills obligations in the economic system. Or it could be sociologically answered with health regarded as a condition appropriate to the social norms and cultural traditions that shape the individual's outlook and values.

In this book, an attempt is made to resolve this multiplicity of views into a small number of distinctive concepts, and to clarify these ideas. In addition, the impact of different notions of the health-illness continuum on policies affecting community health and community health programs is considered.

This interest in the analysis of the idea of health is the result of questions and perplexities that emerged during twenty years of professional nursing practice in settings of acute care and community health. From time to time, situations arose in which the usual signs and symptoms of disease were absent. Yet in some indeterminate sense illness was undeniably present. Pain, debility, extreme incapacitating lethargy appeared in the condition of some patients without being announced by the usual overt failures of health. While classic signs and symptoms of illness on the whole provide effective bases for admission to or discharge from hospitals, experience in community health practice provides numerous instances of "illness" that could not meet these classical standards. What of the 36-year-old mother of six and grandmother of two who is altogether devoid of these hospital standards of illness but who is so enervated, so apathetic that she is utterly unable to perform her customary roles in her home? What is the criterion of health by which this symptomatically well person is appraised as ill?

Cases of this type challenged the adequacy of the textbook criteria of health not because these criteria were false but because in such situations they seemed to fail in their function and left the question of health undecided. Out of such perplexities arose the hypothesis that the traditional generic concept of health can be analyzed into subdivisions of several different kinds of health. Indeed, it soon appeared that it must be so subdivided if we are to deal adequately with the different forms that illness or failure of health may take.

In all its varied meanings, health was recognized as having one formal significance, namely, one extreme of the health-illness continuum. But analysis showed that the gradation of this health-illness continuum may be interpreted in four different and significant ways. To each of these corresponded a certain concept of health care. These were finally integrated into what are here called four distinct models of health.

Four terms have been selected which are used repeatedly and which have varying interpretations in different contexts. To avoid misinterpretation, the following paragraphs state the specific sense in which the terms are used in this book.

Paideia is a Greek word recurring frequently in the literature of ancient Greek philosophy. No single English word can translate it and retain the full, profound meaning of the Greek word. Therefore, the Greek term, closely following the usage in Werner Jaeger's great work *Paideia: The Ideals of Greek Culture*, has been retained. The word means, to begin with, art of civilization. It is an art whose objective is the development of that character and qualities of life in which the individual can attain the fullest realization of his potential. Further, paideia seeks the expression of ideals of human nature and conduct that are central to this growth toward self-realization. It is education in its broadest sense: education as the cultivation and communication of the ideals of perfection in mind and body. If health is conceived as comprehensive well-being, as the fullest development of a person's abilities, character, and quality of life, then it may be understood as health-education.

The word *model* within this context pertains to the way in which the continuum or gradation[3] of health-illness is conceived. Health is a comparative term.[4] It is possible to speak of more or less health; of an individual being healthier at one time than at another time, or of one individual being healthier than another. The concept of health, then, involves a "scale" or gradation of health or illness. These gradations assume a different structure according to the human traits or conditions in the gradation. There appear to be different ways of structuring such health-illness gradations. These diverse structures are called "models of the health-illness gradation" or briefly, "models of health."

Medicine is the knowledge and practice dealing with disease and its treatment.[5] As a term characterizing a professional area it may be divided into two subdivisions: the profession of the nurse, and the profession of the physician. As a name characterizing an area of subject matter, the term medicine designates three phases: (1) scientific research into the nature and causes of disease, medical physiology, and epidemiology; (2) the study and practice of treatment of disease; and (3) the study and practice of prevention of disease and maintenance of health. The concept of health promotion is implicit in both prevention of disease and maintenance of health. Historically, nursing has embraced the second and third of the above phases.

Concerning the professional subdivisions of the nurse and the physician, increasing attention has been recently given to the question whether the nurse's profession is in some sense independent from the physician's. The question is not easily answered, for it entails a complex reappraisal of the educational foundation, the range of professional practice authorized by law and professional rule, and the role of the nurse within the culture and community. Significant considerations have been advanced in support of a policy that would open to nurses an expanded scope of practice. These policies still await clear and definitive formulation, but it is apparent already that the present ferment of discussion and self-examination within the profession will give rise to notable reforms. These developments are noted here in place of a final definition of nursing because of this period of flux. Nursing may in the future be viewed as a branch of medicine not ancillary to the practice of the physician.

Risk, as used here, is the probability of an organism developing a condition of disease or other organic or behavioral abnormality. A risk is said to be self-imposed if the causes that tend to bring about the disease or abnormal condition are avoidable and are due to patterns of life chosen and cultivated by the individual.

The analysis of the concept of health is focused on three main themes concerning the profession of nursing: (1) the scope and aims of the practice of nursing, (2) the role and responsibility of nursing in its social context, and (3) the interest of nursing in the quality of life.

The medical care system in this country is concerned especially with acute episodic illnesses and with traumatic conditions that require advanced hospital-based knowledge and skills. Indeed, most nurses spend much of their professional time caring for people who are suffering from such illnesses and accidents.

In recent decades, however, there has been a movement of ideas toward expanding the vista of medical sciences and arts. From this emerging viewpoint, the concerns of nursing go beyond the physiologic conditions of the body. The kind of care needed most often today is related to out-of-hospital settings and conditions associated with chronic degenerative diseases, environmental contaminants, and those that are man-made because of self-imposed risks, such as smoking, sedentary lifestyles, and drug and food abuse. Such risks, writes Marc Lalonde, "and the environment are the principal or important underlying factors in each of the five major causes of death between the ages of one and seventy and . . . unless the environment is changed and the self-imposed risks are reduced, the death rates will not be significantly improved."[6]

This calls for increasing interest on the part of the nurse in the patient's social role, way of life, values, and in general in the patient's place within the social fabric. Indeed, from this viewpoint, nurses would extend their activities beyond the patient so that in addition to the therapy of the ailing, their work would include the maintenance of health and a reform of the social and physical environment. The interest of the nursing profession may thus become enlarged to include basic social reforms aimed at the ideal of the healthy mind in a healthy body.

In their most general aspect, human traits are either inherited or the result of the interaction between the individual and the environment. Health is thus individually a product of environment and, consequently, the effective care and maintenance of health must involve appropriate controls over the environment. In this light, the practice of nursing unavoidably includes a concern with the physical, social, and cultural milieu of the patient. In this connection, the emphatic observations of the U.S. Public Health Service are noteworthy:

> Although causal relationships have not been demonstrated, there are well established associations between rising unemployment or generally poor economic conditions and increases in child abuse, crime, and among some groups, increases in suicides and homicides. These factors affect not only the person's psychological equilibrium but possibly his ability to resist disease as well. One theory suggests that disturbances

within a person's cultural and social setting generate psychological stress, upset the normal hormonal patterns of the individual, and thereby make him more susceptible to disease.[7]

Although these views are still not widely held, they are nevertheless not new. In the writings of Rudolf Virchow, the "father of pathology," there is already a recognition of health rather than merely disease as the focal concern of medicine and, in consequence, medicine itself ceases to be confined to the technical phases of medical physiology and therapy. Medicine, as he said, whatever else it may be, is also a social science. It is from this viewpoint that he proposed his three guiding principles for medicine: (1) the health of the people is a matter of direct concern; (2) social and economic conditions have an important effect on health; and (3) steps must be taken to promote health in addition to combating disease, and the measures involved in such action must be social as well as medical.[8] In large measure, this inquiry is concerned with the implications and significance of the principles of Virchow. In a way it explores the concept of nursing as a social science, as the knowledge and skill for the attainment of the best quality of life available.

Conventional or traditional forms of medical intervention cannot cope with all of today's health problems. In keeping with Virchow's advice, the health professions must look to wider social horizons to achieve adequate health care in modern society. The following comment by a government agency is illustrative: "The annual carnage on our highways generates costly demands on the health care system but the behavior of the individual behind the wheel of a speeding car and the condition of the car and the highway are determined by social, cultural and economic factors that have little direct involvement with the health professions."[9]

Such social reorientation of the health professions raises questions concerning the extent of government action required for the resolution of such problems. In addition, certain policies regarding education and the environment are entailed in further advances in individual and community health. Accordingly, nursing practice is seen as involving the cultivation of "self-care," the dissemination of knowledge concerning disease prevention, the instruction of the patient in the maintenance and promotion of health, the motivation of the patient for active application of this knowledge, and the cultivation by the patient of life styles and behavior conducive to health. Socially oriented nursing implies environmental policies bearing on the conditions in modern industrial society. It must face the paradoxes of such a society in which desirable social ends are sought by disruptive and pernicious means. We are seeing increasingly persuasive evidence linking a range of human diseases to our industrial society. "Failure to deal with the contamination of our environment could result in serious health consequences whose full effects may not be known for decades to come."[10] Community health services are directed not only at the formulation of broad social policy but at changing social values and enterprises as well.

One aim of this book is to take some first steps toward the development of a theory of health and a philosophy of nursing practice. It is hoped, in addition to any pragmatic professional results, that the inquiry can be of general intellectual interest in the history of ideas and culture.

Chapter 2

NURSING AND MEDICINE

A Historical View

Nursing apparently appears quite late in the historical development of medicine. Fragmentary records of ancient medicine seem to indicate that the medical practitioners of these remote past cultures gave no thought to the kind of therapeutic attention and care that modern nursing provides. The patient's condition was diagnosed by magical or natural means, some treatment was administered by the physician, and the patient was left to the sympathy and attention of lay friends and relatives. This informal care was not in any sense part of medical practice. It was incidental to it and one assumes its existence only by presumption. The historical literature makes no reference to such care of the patient.[1]

It is necessary, of course, to distinguish this sympathetic, informal care of the patient from what is appropriately called nursing care. There are two main lines of distinction: one is concerned with the aim or objective of the care, and the other with its methodology. The sympathetic care, as we may call this type, is passive and largely negative. It provides assistance for the patient to the degree that the patient is helpless and it is guided by empathy and common sense toward the relief of the patient's pain and discomfort. On the other hand, the activity that we designate as nursing care aims not merely at relief from pain but seeks positive objectives in healing and curing the ailment. Furthermore, nursing care, in contrast to sympathetic care, is systematic and bases itself on the best available knowledge concerning the course or natural history of the disease.

In ancient medicine, one can note only two instances of the cultivation of nursing care. One of these is explicitly mentioned in the literature; the other is implicitly indicated. The former appears in ancient India about the first century A.D.[2] The surviving anthology of that period, the Charaka Samhita, refers to a type of medical assistant that is characterized as the "nurse." There seems to be reference to the role of the nurse in Greek medicine of the Hippocratic period. There are some historical indications suggesting that what might be called the medical student or intern in modern literature performed the tasks of systematic nursing care. Apart from these instances, one has to wait for the eighteenth century for the beginnings of modern nursing.

Medicine reached significant developments in ancient Babylonia, India, Greece, and Rome. Throughout the Babylonian literature on medicine, there is no mention or even a sign of any medical or paramedical vocation that we might identify as nursing. It is safe to assume that if there were "nurses," as there seem to have been in ancient India, the various provisions for medicine as written on surviving tablets[3] and the malpractice regulations of the Hammurabi Code would have taken note of it.

The absence of any mention of nursing is significant in light of the fact that extant tablets of law mention numerous details concerning the practice of medicine. The tablets address such topics as bodily parts and diseases associated with them, medicinal properties of plants, and descriptions of techniques of massage, bandaging, poulticing. The Hammurabi Code states, for example, that "if a physician shall make a severe wound with an operating knife and kill a person, or shall open an abscess with an operating knife and destroy the eye, his hands shall be cut off."[4] It is notable that the records indicate a wide interest in public health. The Babylonians were concerned about the sanitary conditions of their cities in order to ensure hygienic settings for the populace. Archeological evidence shows that by 2000 B.C. they had home and town drainage, paved bathrooms, pottery drains, and brick wells.[5] It appears clear that however advanced and closely regulated, Babylonian medicine functioned without the medical role that is assigned to nurses in modern times.

The situation in ancient India was quite different. The relatively high achievement of Indian medicine seemed to have brought with it the establishment of hospitals and the new vocation of trained nurses. It seems that medical training was intensive, systematic, and inspired in part by the Hindu religion.

Young students from the higher castes acquired an elementary knowledge of medicine along with grammar, art, logic, and philoso-phy. The familiarity with basic medical concepts was considered important, even in general education, because of the Hindu teaching that a sound and clean body was necessary to the attainment of a pure heart and mind.[6] Professional study for the practice of medicine lasted seven years. No ancient cultures of this period had achieved extensive knowledge of the internal structures and functions of the body. Indian medicine also functioned within these limitations. Nevertheless, these ancient Indian doctors are credited with being the most skillful surgeons of ancient times. They used medicated wines as anesthetics, had a wide variety of surgical instruments, and were skilled in such procedures as amputation, laparotomy, and Caesarian section.[7]

Historians have speculated that advancements in surgery resulted in the founding of hospitals and both developments led to the need for another category of medical personnel besides the physician. Hence, the nurse appears for the first time in history.

Indian nurses were men, and were acknowledged to have an im-portant contribution to the success of therapy as indicated in excerpts from the Charaka Samhita:

> The Physician, Drugs, Nurse, and Patient constitute an aggregate of Four. Of what virtues each of these should be possessed so as to become causes for the cure of disease should be known. . . . Knowledge of the manner in which drugs should be prepared or compounded for adminis-tration, cleverness, devotedness to the patient waited upon, and purity [of both mind and body] are the four qualifications of the attending Nurse.[8]

The Charaka Samhita in effect details the procedures attached to the nurse's function. It seems that specified places were assigned for the practice of this nursing care. The nurse was expected to be more than a merely loving, devoted attendant. Finally, it is significant that the book explicitly indicates the relationship between the nurse and physician, the nurse acting under the supervision of the doctor. Here is an example of the nursing procedures specified by the Charaka Samhita:

> In the first place a mansion should be constructed. . . . After this should be secured a body of attendants . . . [who are] clever in bathing and washing a patient, well-conversant in rubbing or pressing the limbs; or raising the patient, or assisting him in walking or moving about . . . competent to pound drugs . . . and never unwilling to do any act that they may be commanded to do.[9]

Whether some methods existed to train Indian nurses for these duties is not known but these records do indicate that for the first time, medicine manifested the idea that care—not solely diagnosis and prescription—is part of the medical treatment of the patient.

During the Hippocratic era, which was part of the so-called golden age of ancient Greece, physicians who treated the sick in their homes also recognized the need for skilled attendants rather than merely untrained family members. Since medical education included apprenticeship training, these "medical students" cared for their teachers' patients, carried out their instructions, and performed the treatments. As stated in one of the Hippocratic writings, the physician is to "choose out those who have already been admitted to the mysteries of the art. . . . He is there also to prevent those things escaping notice that happen in the intervals between visits. Never put a layman in charge of anything, otherwise if a mischance occurs the blame will fall on you."[10] In other words, Greek physicians used experienced "medical students" to "nurse" their patients. These students, in order to act responsibly, had to progress to the point in their training where they understood the nature of the illness, the signs and symptoms that would indicate progress or worsening of the patient's condition, and the basis for the prescribed treatment. They apparently exercised discretionary judgment in extending or modifying the physician's regimen in his absence.[11] In short, increased knowledge led to increased responsibilities at the bedside, a situation that has occurred in twentieth-century nursing practice.

Roman medicine had no doctors who matched the caliber of the Greeks until the third century b.c., when Greek physicians began emigrating to Rome. While they used Greek medical writings and learned from the Greek physicians, Roman physicians never expanded upon Greek medical ideas and, therefore, never developed independently of them. They apparently ignored the Greek use of the trained "medical student" in caring for the sick at home. The Greek physician Galen (129–199 a.d.) was preeminent in the Roman Empire and had written the most authoritative medical treatises of the time. Nevertheless, there is no mention in his writings of nurses or comparable roles in medical practice.

Apparently, no nursing care was provided for the Roman legions. The Roman soldiers, even in battles fought close to home, were left to care for and to dress each others' wounds. As there were no field hospitals, the Roman soldier was made as comfortable as possible in nearby homes under the care of lay persons. It was not until military expeditions traveled far from Rome that the care of the sick and wounded became more formalized. When a series of field hospitals was established at strategic points, trained physicians were introduced but it is likely that untrained personnel cared for the soldiers.

The Roman Empire is said to have reached its zenith during 100–180 A.D. Then gradually, over centuries, Roman political and economic life deteriorated. There were increases in the degree of official corruption; a series of incompetent leaders controlled the government; formerly independent farmers became sharecroppers on wealthy estates or migrated to towns and cities; high taxes and inflation discouraged progress in business and commerce. In short, "internal causes had weakened the state and left it exposed on every front."[12] The impact of this weakening of Roman society had its effect on medicine. Soon after the death of Galen in 199 A.D., medical research declined almost to nonexistence. There was a resulting decline of standards for medical practice. Organized, systematic criticism and modification of traditional practice was not encouraged. For centuries after Galen's death, his works were regarded as being all one needed to know about medicine. The more stable Eastern empire was able to preserve ancient Greek and Roman medical writings, which would later be returned to the West by the Mohammedans.

As regards literature and philosophy, there remained very little of that ferment that was characteristic of Roman society even as late as the third century. Because of this intellectual and artistic inactivity, the centuries immediately following (400–1000 A.D.) came to be known as the Dark Ages. The barbarians, who began major invasions of the empire after 400 A.D., had to assimilate the Roman culture before they improved it, a process which took centuries and was not completed until 1500 A.D.

During the growth and subsequent decline of the Roman civilization the new religion, Christianity, was increasing in strength. By 700 A.D., the Roman church was, for the most part, all that remained of the empire.[13]

Christian doctrine emphasized three basic principles: brotherhood, equality before God, and pacifism. This doctrine was interpreted by its followers as placing a higher value on the moral and spiritual qualities of life than on the intellectual and physical aspects of the body. One was to live a moral life in this world in order to achieve everlasting life in the kingdom of heaven. One could live a moral life by working among the sick and the poor. Christians attempted to assist those in distress through humanitarian work, which was viewed as pleasing to God. Thus, in caring for the sick, reactions to the effects of disease, normally viewed as disgusting and trying, were overcome by this particular kind of determination and dedication.

With the church steadily growing in wealth and power, a large percentage of its money was alloted for spiritual as well as charitable purposes.[14] Along with the building of churches, hospitals and xenodochia were established. They were accommodations for the poor, the orphaned, and fatigued and infirm travelers. But Christian humanitarian dedication was adverse to science. In this climate, the weak tradition of nursing descendant from ancient times could not survive. These monastic services to the ailing travelers and pilgrims amounted to a return to primitive sympathetic care without the guidance and professional training of the Indian or Hippocratic "nurse." As we have seen, the idea of a particular place for the care of the sick did not originate with the Christian church. The Indians developed hospitals and the Romans had their military establishments. But Christianity "united the humanitarian efforts of individuals and gave a collective character to charity. Christians preached care of the sick and built numerous institutions on a scale never before mentioned in the history of civilization."[15]

Historical accounts of the Dark Ages and medieval period take note of the founding of hospitals by bishops, kings, and wealthy laity. In all areas of Western Europe, men and women personally ministered to the sick. Church encouragement of these humanitarian efforts did not lead to progress in either medicine or nursing. The Christian hospitals provided loving care but apparently not scientific medicine. They were vehicles for expressing Christian sentiment and humanitarian dedication, which were viewed as virtues far exceeding the virtues of scientific knowledge. The Christian churchmen reacted against the classical sciences like medicine. There were instances when Christians were disciplined for studying such "pagan" subjects. With church emphasis on the cultivation of the spirit and the brightest people choosing to join the church, the secular practice of medicine built on Galen almost disappeared by the sixth century A.D. What took its place were Roman and German superstitious practices, Christian faith healing, and folk medical practices, all combined in varying degrees according to the particular time and place.[16]

With the decline of central Roman authority and a new wave of invasions, like those of the Vikings, the old Roman order was succeeded by a feudal society. Life was spent in rural isolation and self-sufficiency. Most people lived in small villages, usually connected with a manor. They rarely saw anyone from outside their own areas, so everything eaten, worn, spun, and milled was made or grown in the village and manor house. During this period, the clergy were the only group to maintain some semblance of medical practice. While many did not have the education to understand the more complicated treatises of Greek and Roman medicine, they did compile Latin summaries of treatments found useful in daily practice. Notes dealing with the uses of herbs, leeches, and folk medical remedies have been found on the flyleaves of their books. Such medical practices were of an elementary nature and generally limited to monastic infirmaries. The few monks who had some scientific medical skills acquired these before they took their monastic vows. The monastery itself was inimical to the cultivation of scientific medicine and consequently, one may suppose, inhibited the development of nursing during this age. In time, medical practice among laymen by the monastic physician outside of the monasteries was discouraged by the church because it was viewed as neglecting religious duties of a more spiritual nature.

As we have seen, in ancient times nursing care was practiced primarily by men. However, at this time, 1100–1400 A.D., women entered the field in large numbers. This was brought about by the growth of certain secular orders that began to establish women's auxiliaries dedicated to the care of the sick. When St. Francis of Assisi (1182–1226) founded the order of friars who practiced their Christian mission outside monasteries, his friend Clarissae organized an affiliated order of women to help them. These so-called Poor Clares mended the friars' clothes, took care of their church, and ministered to the sick who needed special care. Subsequently, another female order with similar interests was established in 1296 and was named the Oblates of Florence. The entry of women into these orders rendering devoted care to the sick was very far from signifying the emergence of some kind of nursing profession. It is doubtful that the Poor Clares and others like them had any scientific medical training, although there is reason to believe that the Oblates of Florence were given some systematic medical instruction in preparation for their nursing vocation. In any case, medical education and practice had been allowed to decline. Medical instruction was based almost exclusively on incorrectly translated excerpts of treatises. Hardly any original classical works in medicine were still in circulation.

It was not until the ninth century that Europe saw the restoration of scientific medicine, which occurred at the Salerno School of Medicine. In the next three centuries, the Salerno School grew into Europe's foremost medical center. In time, other centers of medical learning appeared, some of which developed into great universities. The layman interested in entering the medical profession now had a rich resource for learning.

Formal education at these university centers rapidly increased the number of graduate medical doctors. The practice of these lay, university-educated physicians at first tended to focus on patients among the well-to-do upper classes. The ailing poor derived little benefit from these early advances in the profession and still depended on such medical care as was provided by religious and secular church orders. Guilds of medical practitioners began to appear and promised to consolidate medical advances by regulating the practice of the profession. Unfortunately, the women's auxiliaries who might have extended these benefits to the poorer classes were no longer available. Rigorous restraints imposed by the church on the practices of these orders, as well as the challenges of the Reformation, led to the erosion of these useful "nursing" orders. Members of these orders might have served as professional nurses, but history denied them this opportunity. In time, a number of historical trends and agencies transformed the hospitals from religious to secular institutions. The newly evolved hospitals felt the impact of the decline of these "nursing" orders. Without them, there was no source of hospital personnel for the care of the patients at any but the most primitive level. Gradually, the idea that care of the sick was a valuable humanitarian pursuit was lost. It became disagreeable work unsuitable for any woman of refinement and intelligence. It became work identified with the lowest classes—people who were poor and ignorant. No corrective for this condition appeared, so that even as late as the nineteenth century the care of the sick was in a deplorable state. Nothing replaced the religious orders and much of the care was haphazard.[17]

The modern medical profession inevitably recognized the need for reform. More and more physicians began to write about the importance of quality attendant care in the recovery of the patient. As early as 1765, in an article entitled "Infirmier" in *The French Encyclopedia*, the author states that while all persons are not adapted for the low and repugnant functions of nursing, "heads of hospitals ought to be difficult to please, for the lives of patients may depend on choice of applicants."[18]

The German physician Franz May affirmed that poor nursing care "was a major cause of hospital mortality and that the service must be improved in the interest of public health."[19] By 1782, in connection with his lectures at a Mannheim hospital, he published a manual on nursing that was used for the instruction and guidance of attendants there. Years later, in 1801, he established nursing courses at Heidelberg.

At this time, a number of hospitals maintained by religious orders were still in existence despite a trend in Protestant countries toward the elimination of church-related institutions. These religious hospitals were managed and staffed by religious orders like the Beguines and Sisters of Charity. Many physicians of the period held the members of the religious orders in high regard and characterized them as pious, devoted, honest, clean, and organized.[20] This high reputation of the religious nursing orders resulted in their being preferred over the secular nursing personnel in the hospitals. Contemporary professional comment on these secular nurses indicates marked scorn for their alleged irregularity, undependability, and generally low character.[21] The direct remedy for this marked inferiority of the secular nurses would have been the establishment of professional educational institutions for nurses. However, the availability of the highly dependable religious orders made the need for reform less urgent. In consequence, the establishment of effective institutions for nursing education was delayed.

The revival of a vigorous nursing vocation was stimulated by the recognition of a medical role for the nurse. The continuing link of hospital nursing to religious vocation was a significant factor in this new growth of nursing as a medical role for women. A focal point in this development was the formation of a deaconess order by Pastor Theodore Fliedner. This new religious order was centered in the German town of Kaiserswerth, where the motherhouse came to be established. The new German order served as a model for other establishments. The famed Quaker and social reformer Elizabeth Fry, having visited the order in Kaiserswerth, was instrumental in the organization of a similar establishment in England. This was the Institute of Nursing in London. Although it was primarily an educational institution, its students were designated as the Protestant Sisters of Charity and, in fact, functioned as members of a Protestant religious order similar to the German order of deaconesses. They were sent to Guy's Hospital to gain experience in nursing. What little scientific training they received there was gotten by casual instructions from the physicians, for the staff attendants in the hospital, it seems, had no systematic medical training. The students, upon completion of their program, were expected to do what today is called private duty nursing in the home.

Improved education and training procedures for nurses were fostered by the other religious orders. For example, the Anglican Church established programs for training nurses in various London hospitals. This educational and nursing program was administered under the so-called Community of St. John's House. This community was instrumental in recruiting nurses to serve under Florence Nightingale in the Crimean War.

Florence Nightingale was a devoutly religious person, but she did not think that the education and training of nurses and the practice of nursing should be left to the management of religious orders. Instead, she fostered secular scientific education for nursing. Some medical men and social reformers had already contended that more than sympathy and devotion were needed for effective nursing. The modern nurse, they held, needed to be scientifically trained. Nightingale's Crimean experiences convinced her of the correctness of this view. She saw nursing as concerned with both health and illness. The art of nursing, she believed, provided the best means for the restoration or preservation of health, and prevention or cure of disease and injury. For Nightingale, nursing was an art—but this art was not spontaneous. It could be cultivated only on the basis of organized practical and scientific training.[22]

In the hospitals, she felt that the ward sisters and physicians should teach the nurses to know the symptoms of diseases, the causes of such symptoms, and the reasons for specific types of therapy. In addition, she proposed starting schools where both theoretical knowledge and clinical experience would be provided for the nursing recruits. The first of these schools was established in 1860 at St. Thomas's Hospital in London. The students were taught the principles of hygiene and sanitation and to care for the sick.[23] About fifteen years after the first school was founded, most hospitals in England had at least one "Nightingale" nurse, that is to say, a product of Nightingale's program of training. Many other hospitals instituted their own training schools based on the Nightingale program. The nurses trained under this system were soon recognized as superior; their discipline was more reliable, and their character and general moral tone gave assurance of their professional dedication.

The professional and social impact of these developments was very extensive. The scientifically trained Nightingale nurses were in great demand throughout the hospital system. Notable improvements were achieved in the hospital care of the sick. These recognized professional accomplishments aroused wide interest and attracted a better class of women to the nursing profession.

The high accomplishments were certainly not achieved overnight. Nursing evidently did not enjoy a socially high status. The nurses' living conditions in the hospitals were inferior, the hours of labor unduly long. In short, the condition of nurses was no better than that of the hard pressed and deprived laboring classes. In 1868, when Dr. Samuel Gross, president of the American Medical Association, made his innovative proposal for the scientific education of nurses, it was far from a proposal for the improvement of the social and professional status of nurses. Gross stressed that it was necessary to have well-trained, well-instructed nurses working with intelligent and skilled physicians because the physicians' efforts were of little avail unless seconded by an intelligent and devoted nurse.[24]

The first attempts to institute such scientific education in the United States were halting and had little influence on the nurses' quality of life. The scientific education of nurses begun one hundred years ago at the New England Hospital for Women and Children may have improved the nurses' skills, but it did nothing to relieve the arduous conditions of their lives. The educational program was brief and altogether subordinate to the demands of the nurses' jobs in the wards. They were expected to work in the wards from 5:30 A.M. to 9:00 P.M. and to sleep in rooms near the wards so they could handle emergencies during the night.[25] The situation was not much improved when a second program of nursing education was instituted in 1873 at Bellevue Hospital in New York City. Many years passed before it was recognized that the professional advancement of nurses with regard to education presupposes a radical reform of their working conditions and status.

New Horizons

Improvements in the scientific education and working conditions of nurses eventually provoked questions concerning the nurse's status, as well as the technical authority of the services the nurse renders.

What is the status of the nurse? The issues precipitated by this question have engendered wide controversy in the nursing profession. Whatever side is taken, it is essential to bear in mind the historical road that brought the profession to its present level. As we have seen, the history of nursing is also a history of the advances in the scientific training of the nurse. This professional education emerged as the technical, professional requirements for the nurse's role were recognized. With the advancement in professional education, there came certain refinements in the service the nurse performed. The key to an adequate appreciation of any future reform in the character of the service and professional skill of the nurse depends, therefore, on a clear grasp of the nurse's role in the total health cycle.

What is here called the health cycle is the succession of stages of activity from the initial recognition of an illness to the restoration of health. In very brief outline, we can distinguish five traditional stages:

1. Presence of illness or disability is recognized by its signs and symptoms.
2. The illness or disability is diagnosed as due to specified causes.
3. A specific remedy or therapy is prescribed.
4. The therapy is administered by the physician or surrogate (as in surgery, for example).
5. In the absence of the physician
   A. in the case of a patient not incapacitated by the illness: the patient administers the remedy or therapy.
   B. in the case of an incapacitated patient (bedridden in a hospital): the prescribed remedy or therapy is administered, the patient is continually observed, unexpected modifications in the patient's condition are interpreted and treated, the patient is instructed in continuing the therapy at an eventual self-administered level.

The foregoing sequence of events presents the formal schema of intervention in illness. Needless to say, in the actual history of illness and its treatment, this schema is modified by details and by the varying duration of the different stages. Some stages may be repeated, but the general pattern and sequence will be followed. This outline is introduced here only as a device for clarifying the role of the nurse and the relation of that role to the role of the physician.

The preeminent role in stages 2, 3, and 4 is performed by the physician while the role in stage 5B is performed by the nurse. The nurse may also perform a significant role in stages 2, 3, and 4, as assistant to the physician (as do nurse practitioners when viewed within the context of the health cycle), but the role designated in Stage 5B is the preeminent traditional role of the nurse.

It is important to recognize that the role designated in stage 5B is an indispensable part of the cycle. Without it, the physician's role would be largely nullified. In this sense, therefore, the role in stage 5B completes or fulfills the role performed by the physician. This indispensable role is the role of the nurse.

The nursing role in this cycle involves a considerable range of discretionary judgment and reflection. The doctor issues orders; the nurse is required to carry them out. By the nature of the nursing role, the nurse must carry orders out critically in light of the continued evaluation of the patient's condition and the patient's specific environmental situation. This is not a job for an automaton, mechanically following the doctor's orders. The nurse knows the intent of the orders, thinks about them, follows the general order but takes his or her own findings into account. This cannot be done without considerable scientific "medical" education and training.

Large numbers of nurses in this country have become increasingly dissatisfied with the functions they have been required to perform on their jobs. The burden of routine tasks and the emphatic precedence enjoyed by the doctors in relation to the nurse's duties are probably major factors in the restive professional discontent among nurses. This situation, as well as the continued inadequate salary scales, has tended to underscore the seemingly inferior and subordinate status of the nurse. In the eyes of many contemporary nurses, the discontent tends to be focused on the professional subservience of the nurse to the doctor. They feel, accordingly, that both salary scales and public esteem would be elevated if the nurse could achieve a significant measure of independence from the doctor.

The increase in the complexity of modern health care and a concomitant advancement and intensification of the theoretical education and technical training of the nurse have resulted in some questions and quandaries concerning the scope of discretion exercised by the nurse. These developments have also resulted in the nurse having a considerable share in knowledge normally imparted to the physician. Thus, unavoidable questions have arisen as to the role of the nurse in the delivery of health care, with a growing trend toward an independent, discretionary status for the nurse. This has led to the emergence of independent nursing practitioners, community health practitioners, psychiatric clinical specialists, and so on.

At this point, the controversy becomes confused. Proposals for professional recognition of such specialty groups (in so-called expanded roles) are, in fact, not pertinent to the reform of the nurse's role. Their aim is *not* the improvement of the role defined above in stage 5B. What they do propose is the design and establishment of an altogether new role. It is not clear where advocates of these new professional roles would place them in the health cycle, but they clearly do not belong strictly at stage 5B. It is conceivable that a particular individual trained to perform the nursing role at stage 5B might decide to abandon that role and seek a career in the proposed new roles of independent nurse practitioner, community health practitioner, and so on. But such decisions to seek a new career affect only the individual person involved. They do not in any way affect the design and performance of the nurse's role as stipulated in the foregoing schema.

This is not said to denigrate the professional movement toward the institution of those new roles. These innovations may prove highly desirable in the future development and extension of health care. They may be welcome as providing alternative careers for graduates of basic nursing programs. These new careers may even prove more rewarding emotionally and financially.

Nevertheless, such developments cannot alter the demand for the performance of the traditional nursing role. Someone with the appropriate qualifications must perform that role, as that role is an indispensable part of the health cycle. The issues in the controversy, therefore, are complex. The debate spreads over at least two questions:

1. Shall the new roles be given general recognition and how shall these new roles be designed?
2. How shall the nursing role of stage 5B be redesigned to make optimal use of the nurse's technical skills and, at the same time, clarify the nurse's status as that of a highly trained professional?

The succeeding chapters are, in effect, varieties of world views open to adoption by the nurse.

Conclusion

Since its beginnings in ancient times, nursing has developed a close dependence on the art and science of the physician. The nurse was the handmaiden of the physician, with no more than the rudimentary knowledge of medicine sufficient for this ancillary, dependent role. In time, the inadequacies of the lay nurse led to a recognition of the need for formal training and eventually to the development of schools for secular, scientific nursing education. This was the beginning of a trend that culminated in the present policy, which seeks to parallel the scientific education of the nurse with the general developments in the science and technology of medicine.

The historical motivation for this scientific education was the improved effectiveness of the traditional role of the nurse. But an incidental and unavoidable consequence was a transformation of the nurse's outlook. With advanced scientific training came a critical awareness of medical situations and the doctor's decisions. Questions arose in the minds of many nurses concerning the status of the nurse, the scope of discretion in the nurse's practice, and the range of subordination of the nursing role to the role of the physician.

The "nurse liberation movement" provides some answers to these questions, but the impact of this movement on the traditional nursing role is not clear. The movement encourages the development of new roles for nurses with advanced scientific education such as the independent nurse practitioner. This, however, does not affect the character and need for that indispensable nursing role cited above under 5B in the health cycle. Regardless of the new careers for nurses, there still remains the need for people with appropriate education to fulfill this necessary role in 5B. There still remain urgent questions as to how this role may be made more effective.

What we need is a clarification of the professional duties of the traditional nurse. For example, how can this nursing role be made more effective and efficient in light of the technical education and training of the nurse? One solution to this problem is to eliminate the housekeeping and sanitation functions still associated with nursing. Requiring the same person who performs the highly technical functions of the trained nurse to also perform the menial, relatively unskilled tasks of housekeeping tends to obscure the status of the nurse. The confusion of roles prevents many patients from perceiving the nurse as an educated, scientific professional.

Chapter 3

HEALTH AS PAIDEIA

A nurse or physician caring for a patient who complains of fever and productive cough may be seen as confronted by a disease or by an individual human being whose normal life has become disrupted. These alternatives are not mutually exclusive. Nevertheless, in the eyes of many nurses and physicians the former alternative is more effectively and efficiently handled through the exclusion of the latter. The patient's complaints are identified in the diagnosis as arising from some irregularity or disorder of a specific subsystem of the larger physiological organization of the body. The examination as well as the treatment thus becomes narrowed to those particular features of the body. It may be argued that no subsystem is independent of the organism as a whole. But the fact remains that modern medicine has successfully treated certain diseases, such as infectious diseases, as if the locus of the disease was isolable from the rest of the organism. For example, a bronchial infection may be treated without regard to urine pH, sugar levels in the blood, or degree of stress experienced by the patient.

On the other hand, when the patient's complaint is seen within the context of his total life, the task of the nurse and physician is enlarged and altered in important ways. Interest comes to be focused on the health of the patient and this health may involve much more than the recovery from some specific disorder or the relief from some specific pain.

The present trend in the nurse's and the physician's education emphasizes the anatomy and physiology of organ systems and the pathophysiologic changes that can result in disease. The focus on pathophysiology has tended to shift emphasis away from concern with the individual who happens to be sick to concern with that person's disease. This has resulted in narrowing the scope of contemporary medicine as compared with ancient Greek medicine.

While it is highly desirable that medical science cultivate technological developments and intensive specialized knowledge and skill, this should not eclipse the value of broader and in a sense more fundamental objectives of medicine. This role of medicine transcends the diagnosis and treatment of disease or medical therapeutics. Its ultimate concern is with ideals of health and its preservation. In this role the nurse and the medical doctor become the cultivators and teachers of certain attitudes toward life.

The Ideal of Health in Hippocratic Medicine

It is notable that early Greek medicine in the era of Hippocrates viewed the treatment of disease and dysfunction as inseparable from what it conceived as the entire nature of man. Man was viewed as a part of nature, which was seen as an organic, teleological system. An opposed outlook, the mechanistic conception of nature, later came to dominate the development of physiology and medicine.

The teleological, holistic conception of nature and its role in medical thought was a well-established tradition by the time of Plato. This view finds a vivid expression in the *Charmides* of Plato. The following is typical: "an ailment of the eyes or head cannot be cured without reference to the whole body."[1] In other words, a physician cannot adequately treat a part without giving consideration to the whole. This interpretation of Hippocratic thought treats this organismic outlook as applicable especially to the relation of a part of the human body to the order or system of the body as a whole. In light of another interpretation, Hippocratic medical thought was based on the doctrine of an organic, teleological relation between the human body and the order of the universe of which it is a part. This point is reflected in the *Phaedrus* of Plato.

Socrates: And do you think that you can know the nature of the soul intelligently without knowing the nature of the universe?

Phaedrus: If Hippocrates the Asclepiad is to be trusted, even the nature of the body cannot be understood without that sort of inquiry.[2]

These two interpretations are, of course, not inconsistent. Both express an underlying teleological conception of nature with which Plato's philosophy was in full agreement.

Greek medical thought of the Hippocratic era arrived at this point through the influence of early nature philosophy. Under the influence of its teleological, organismic philosophy of nature, ancient medicine was oriented toward broad social objectives through which, without neglecting the relief and cure of the ailing, it made significant contributions to its age. Among these phases of Hippocratic medicine, the following are important:

1. *Its emergence as a significant methodical empirical science under the influence of Ionian "nature" philosophy; the development of the idea of the physical nature of man as inseparable from the nature of the environment.* The Hippocratics applied the empiric methods learned from the nature philosophers to the scientific observation of the body and its processes.[3] For example, they made careful, systematic observations of the patients and their surroundings. A patient's appearance, behavior, signs, symptoms, moods, excretions, secretions were checked with specific attention paid to the organ or part that was deranged. The patient, family, and friends were interviewed. The condition of the physical environment was noted. All findings were recorded in the form of a case history.[4]

The Hippocratics learned to generalize from specific cases. By noting similarities and differences among patients they tried to explain interrelationships among signs and symptoms. They used metaphors and analogies in order to make their explanations clearer (for example, the lungs acted like bellows and the heart like a pump). They always returned to the bedside to make sure that their explanations fitted reality and that their treatments produced results.

Since the Hippocratics saw man as part of a larger whole, they were very interested in man in relation to the physical environment. They knew that winds, climate, air, seasons, and geographic locale all affected man's health.[5]

2. *The extensive popularization (humanization) of medical knowledge; making popular health education a part of the overall interest of medicine.*[6] Medicine was not esoteric in this era. Physicians gave public lectures on health, disease, and related topics. They wrote medical treatises intended for use by the layman. They spoke of the kinds of problems faced in practice in order to stimulate people to maintain or restore their health and to ensure their cooperation in treatment.

3. *The rise of the idea of health as a virtue to be cultivated on a parallel with moral virtue.* This is one of the most interesting and significant ideas emerging from the ancient Greek philosophy of medicine. The early philosophers who wrote before the time of Plato were the first to use and develop the notion "nature of the universe." This may seen like a simple, commonplace notion but it is in fact a revolutionary innovation in our cultural history.[7] Before the rise of Ionian nature philosophy, Greek culture was dominated by such mysteries as the Orphic religion and other mystical, supernaturalistic influences that saw the world as dark, unintelligible, arbitrary.[8] Man was viewed as being subject to forces that were not understandable because they were not subject to inquiry and investigation. The Ionian philosophers' interest in natural science and a naturalistic philosophy was in conflict with these older mystery religions. These early philosophers looked at the world about them and wanted to know its "nature." In the attempts to answer the questions they raised, they developed naturalistic explanations for their observations.[9] Nature, they said, is order, proportion. It can be conceived as having a fixed, ideal character. The universe and everything in it has fixed characteristics of symmetry, order, proportion that are proper to it. The world and everything in it is seen as striving toward the attainment and maintenance of this proportion. This idea of nature as an ordered system governed by fixed, impersonal principles is rational, orderly, intelligible, and is the antithesis of the outlook of the mystery religions that saw nature as demonic and subject to unpredictable influences.

Seen as a new way of looking at the world, this view of nature had special impact on medical thought. It provided the Hippocratic physicians with a theoretical basis for their conception of health and disease. Health came to be viewed as related to the nature, the intrinsic tendencies, the "natural proportions" of the human body; the human body was conceived as a physical system with a particular structure to be understood in a particular way. Man was subject to certain rules, rules that were appropriate to the *nature* of man. The knowledge of these rules was the most effective way to preserve health or recover from disease.[10]

From this viewpoint, the essential nature of health was equality, harmony, symmetry—properties that constituted order within the physical organism. Thus health became, for the Hippocratics, the standard for physical existence.[11] With man's physical nature viewed as having intrinsic tendencies toward health, to be unhealthy meant that one was less of a man. With normal health originating in the proportion of the parts of the body, this proportion was viewed as the cause of the physical virtues: health, strength, and beauty, which Plato spoke of as parallel to the ethical virtues of the soul.[12]

Physical health became a human virtue, one of the fundamental cultural values worth striving for; once attained, it was the duty of man to live in a way that preserved this virtue of health.[13] Thus health was a *natural* quality—the aim of the intrinsic, natural striving of the body. Medicine itself emerged as the guide of this natural tendency toward the preservation of health.

Public Health in Modern Times: Renaissance of the Ancient Greek Ideal

The achievements of ancient medicine came to be neglected. Medical practice, over a long period of its subsequent history, aimed primarily at the alleviation of pain and the restoration of the patient to his accustomed condition. The idea of health thus became confined to the absence of conspicuous, debilitating signs and symptoms of sickness. Rather than continuing its interest in the education of the public, cultivating within a society sound ideas of personal health, medicine has generally limited its role to that of the individual practitioner who acts only in response to a patient's complaints or inquiries.

In modern times, preventive medicine and public health have reoriented medicine toward a greater interest in the education of the public on the conditions required for the avoidance of sickness through hygiene, sanitation, and the maintenance of a proper environment. This new orientation resulted in turn in a changed idea of health as well-being. This development in medicine was influenced by the intellectual and cultural trends of late eighteenth- and early nineteenth-century Europe.

One of the most important ideas to emerge during the late eighteenth century was the notion of "human perfectibility."[14] Men could, given the proper circumstances, attain a condition of perfection on this earth. They did not have to wait for the state of grace that presumably followed death. This notion, Brinton says, stemmed from the works of both Isaac Newton (1642–1727) and John Locke (1632–1704). Newton disclosed the supreme rationality of nature, whereas Locke exposed the rational structure of man. Thus, nothing was hidden to reason either in nature or in man. Reason could open the way to the indefinite improvement of mankind. This supreme confidence in reason, in science, pervaded the period that came to be called the Enlightenment. For later generations of men, the idea of human perfectibility became a standard by which to formulate plans for social progress. And "Reason could show men how to control their environment and themselves."[15] Locke's view that there are no innate ideas encouraged the tendency over generations to see mind as shaped by the environment. Thus, the kind of environment that surrounded man was of the greatest importance. Where the social environment was corrupt, it had to be reformed; where the physical environment was harsh, it had to be made pleasant.[16] The men and women of the Enlightenment tended to believe that if they could "only work out the proper 'arrangements,' laws, institutions, above all education, human beings will get along together in something pretty close to the good life."[17]

A preeminent instance of this scientific orientation of social philosophy is to be found in Jeremy Bentham (1748–1832). For Bentham, mankind is governed by pain and pleasure.[18] Therefore, a policy is approved according to its tendency to increase or diminish the happiness of the individual or the community in question. In other words, to paraphrase Bentham, the policy is evaluated on the basis of its utility to produce benefit, advantage, pleasure, or happiness to the party whose interest is considered. If the party under consideration is the community in general, then the utility in question is the tendency to produce the happiness of the community. Since the magnitude of the utility of a proposed social action is linked to the magnitude of the pleasure it produces, it is according to Bentham rationally calculable.

The interest of the community is the sum of the interests of the members who compose it.[19] Therefore, the happiness of the community is the happiness of the greatest number of its members. The administration of social policy depends on regulations that, on the whole, ensure the utility of the policy for individual happiness— regulations that make abiding by the desired social action yield pleasure to the individual, whereas the contrary action produces pain. Thus, Bentham's utilitarian philosophy provided a basis for social legislation that its followers claimed to be rationally or scientifically determinable. He provided a large part of the foundation upon which the great sanitary movement of the nineteenth century was built.

Bentham's legal and administrative philosophy was implemented by his followers, the Philosophical Radicals. The most prominent Philosophical Radical who dealt with matters related to the public health in nineteenth-century England was Edwin Chadwick (1800–1890). Despite the resistance offered to his reforms, Chadwick's innovative role and achievements in public health were widely acknowledged in his own time, as the following quotation from the *London Times* of 1854 shows:

> Future historians who want to know what a Commission, a Board whether national or local, a secretary whether working or Parliamentary, a Report, a Secretary of State or almost any other member of our system was in the 19th century, will find the name of Chadwick inextricably mixed up with his inquiries. Should he want to know what a job was in those days he will find a clue to his researches in that ubiquitous name. . . . Ask—who did this? Who wrote that? Who managed that appointment, or ordered that sewer, and the answer is always the same—Mr. Edwin Chadwick.[20]

Chadwick believed that significant conditions of the natural and social environment that affected the health and quality of life of a community could be effectively regulated by legislation and administrative agencies. Thus, radical improvements in health that the individual may not be willing or able to undertake could be achieved by such regulatory measures. Chadwick used his position on various commissions to push for the public health measures he valued: adequate and safe water supplies, adequate drainage systems, and improved conditions for the working classes. He made extensive studies of aspects of social life, such as working conditions, burial practices, sewage disposal, water supply, and general living conditions. His reports formed the basis for legislation that implemented far-reaching environmental reforms that raised the level of individual and group health. For example, in certain working-class groups placed in good sanitary conditions, the annual death rate fell from thirty to thirteen per thousand.

The sanitary movement initiated by Chadwick showed that the severity and often fatal character of disease could be alleviated if the conditions of the environment were appropriate. The sanitary movement brought about radical changes in the social outlook of governmental policy. A new awareness of the importance of government intervention in the management of health was stimulated. It was evident to these reformers that responsibility for large-scale public health measures, like ensuring adequate sewage disposal and safe water supplies, could not be left to the whims of individuals or local governments. There must be centralized responsibility with sufficient power to protect the public health. Thus, administrative mechanisms were advanced that provided a change from local government responsibility to the national. The overall effect was the formulation of minimal acceptable standards implemented nationally for the protection of the public health. The regulatory policies of this reform movement rested on the assumption that government has an interest in and a responsibility for the welfare of individuals, even where those individuals may be indifferent to their well-being. This idea was a new notion in the nineteenth century, contrasting with the previously dominant notion of individual responsibility and self-help.

Apart from the practical benefits that obviously result from public health, anyone interested in this subject in relation to social philosophy would be concerned with some kind of theoretical validation of the aforementioned assumption. Is the intervention of government in public health justifiable? Is the intervention of government in the protection of individual health an assault on individual liberty? Such questions would have to be answered by a political philosophy that can provide a theoretical justification for the extension of government into the private concerns of health. Such theoretical inquiries in political philosophy lie outside the purview of this book. For the present, we are content without a theoretical foundation to pursue public health in the interest of welfare and happiness, however unphilosophical its political foundation may be.

It was the growth of science and the development of the scientific method that was probably the most important event in reorienting medicine. From this new perspective, medicine came to view man more within the context of the natural and social environments. When Pasteur's work put the germ theory of disease on a solid foundation, the growth of bacteriology and immunology was rapid. These sciences fostered a consensus on the origin and transmission of infectious diseases and opened the way for their control in a more rational and accurate manner.[21] Preventive medicine and sanitary science were established on this base. Bacteriologists discovered that microorganisms could cause diseases in man, and that they were found in air, water, food, sewage, and spread by insects, rodents, and man himself. The results of public health measures developed from these findings were dramatic. The control and conquest of infectious diseases added decades to the average life-span because of such measures as improved filtration and disinfection of water supplies, pasteurization of milk, careful control of contact with the sick, and immunization programs. These developments opened up a new direction of medical inquiry and practice, namely social medicine. Medicine could no longer ignore the relation of the person to the conditions of the larger environment.

Combined with interest in the preservation and restoration of salutary environments, these recent extensions of medical science can point to a new creative trend in our culture, toward new priorities in which the quality of life will take precedence over the growth-centered and commodity-centered values that have heretofore marked the rise of our technological civilization. The vast advances of medical science since Hippocrates are not irreconcilable with the revival in modern culture of the ancient Greek ideals of medicine—what Werner Jaeger calls paideia, an intrinsic, pervasive element of the culture, active life, and education of a people.

Conclusion

An ideal of health in ancient Greece during the era of the Hippocratic physicians viewed man in relation to the total environment. The underlying philosophy of modern public health can be viewed as resulting in a renaissance of this ancient Greek ideal of health since both the ancient Greeks and the leaders of the nineteenth-century public health movement, who were products of the Enlightenment:

1.   broke with supernaturalistic tradition—the Greeks with their mystery religions because of the Ionian nature philosophers, and the public health leaders with Christian supernaturalism due to the work of Isaac Newton, John Locke, Jeremy Bentham, and the advances in science;
2.   sought naturalistic explanations for the rules of health and the causes of disease;
3.   looked beyond the physiology of the body and included the environment in theories of disease causation; and
4.   viewed the preservation of health as a fundamental value.

It is hoped that a return to the ideal of health that embraces the total human condition will result in the view that a normal healthy mind in a normal healthy body should be a fundamental aim of our culture—an aim of health as paideia.

Chapter 4

FOUR MODELS OF HEALTH

On the basis of tentative investigations of the relevant literature, the various conceptions and ideas of health can be resolved into four distinctive types: (1) clinical model, (2) role-performance model, (3) adaptive model, and (4) eudaimonistic model. Each of these models can be defined by the way the extremes of the health-illness continuum are characterized.

Clinical Model. Health-extreme: absence of signs or symptoms of disease or disability as identified by medical science; illness-extreme: conspicuous presence of these signs or symptoms.

Role-Performance Model. Health-extreme: performance of social roles with maximum expected output; illness-extreme: failure in performance of role.

Adaptive Model. Health-extreme: the organism maintains flexible adaptation to the environment, interacts with environment with maximum advantage; illness-extreme: alienation of the organism from environment, failure of self-corrective responses.

Eudaimonistic Model. Health-extreme: exuberant well-being; illness-extreme: enervation, languishing debility.

The figure that follows, the Health-Illness Continuum, depicts these models diagrammatically.

An analysis of these four concepts of health was done through an examination of the representative literature. The clinical model was

THE HEALTH-ILLNESS CONTINUUM

	Health	Illness
Clinical Model	Absence of signs or symptoms	Conspicuous presence of signs or symptoms
Role-Performance Model	Maximum expected performance	Total failure in performance
Adaptive Model	Flexible adaptation to environment	Total failure in self-corrective response
Eudaimonistic Model	Exuberant well-being	Enervation, languishing debility

explored as implicitly represented in much of contemporary medical practice. The role-performance model was studied through some of the writings of Talcott Parsons and others. The study of the adaptive model focused on the writings of René Dubos, and the examination of the eudaimonistic model of health focused on the writings of Abraham H. Maslow.

Each of the four models of health bears a distinctive relation to social policy regarding nursing and health care. They direct community health policy toward different objectives. The clinical model would enhance funding of categorical disease programs aimed at treating specific medical disorders and disabilities after they have already appeared in the population. This is the situation that presently exists. The role-performance model in its bearing on public health policy would result in more programs in the occupational health sector. The adaptive model would encourage the public health expert to ferret out new conditions detrimental to health. The eudaimonistic model would foster community health programs geared toward fulfilling the basic human needs as described by Maslow and associated with physical and social welfare, safety, and self-fulfillment. This would mean a more comprehensive approach to health, cutting across the traditional boundaries separating the fields of health, education, and individual and community welfare.

The next four chapters seek to make explicit the concepts of health that have emerged in the course of modern history.

Medicine has been described as "the department of knowledge and practice dealing with disease and its treatment." In this context, the term "disease" is usually taken to refer to a disease entity, a morbid physical condition identified by its syndrome of signs and symptoms. The term can be understood to mean something more general, namely, any condition of the body-mind more or less seriously out of health. In the *Oxford English Dictionary*, the term "disease" is defined as "a condition of the body or some part or organ of the body, in which its functions are disturbed or deranged." This conception is, however, implicitly dependent on the idea of sound and normal functioning, in other words, on the idea of the healthy body.

The idea of health plays a central, directive role in every phase of medicine: therapeutic, preventive, public health, and social medicine. The importance of clarifying the idea of health and of distinguishing various conceptions of health is evident in light of the foregoing. The idea of health defines the objectives of medicine (understood in its most general sense) and different conceptions of health direct the nurse's practice and the physician's practice toward different objectives.

In the following discussions of each of the four models of health, the exposition of each distinct idea is followed immediately by an interpretive analysis and, whenever possible, by a critical appraisal. The ideas are explored immediately on presentation. By following each separate idea with its analysis and criticism, the impact of the interpretation and critique upon the idea becomes clear and vivid.

Chapter 5

CLINICAL MODEL

Most people who consult a physician are in pain or are experiencing some more or less acute abnormal condition of the body-mind. The responsive physician seeks to alleviate or eliminate the pain and to free the patient of the derangements and malfunctionings of his organs that constitute the illness or contribute to it. From one point of view, the focus of medical practice thus becomes primarily the elimination of morbid physical or mental conditions and the relief from any concomitant pain. When this relief is attained and the symptoms of disease are no longer present in the body or mind, medical therapy has completed its task. The patient is said to be restored to "health." Health is thus conceived as the absence of disease, a concept that is here called the clinical model of health.

This view of health as the absence of disease is due in large part to the mechanistic outlook that has dominated the development of the biomedical sciences since the seventeenth century. In a sense, contemporary medicine is a product of the mechanistic concept of man. For, in all sciences that comprise medical knowledge, such as anatomy, physiology, biochemistry, the method of mechanistic analysis has been a central theme in their development. Medical knowledge must of course be organized in a way that would guide medical practice. This means a concentration on the study of such aspects of people as their physical structure, physiologic functions, and biochemistry. These biological and physical sciences were based on the method of mechanistic analysis.

A most important result of this method was the emergence of man as a physico-chemical mechanism, or, as the eighteenth-century French physician and philosopher La Mettrie said, *L'Homme-Ma-*

chine. Just as La Mettrie mechanized the idea of man in his notion of man-machine, so his contemporary Paul d'Holbach in *The System of Nature* later mechanized the universe in his concept of nature. One vast mechanism constituted the cosmos as well as man. From this perspective, the physician sees the patient primarily as a physiochemical system. The system functions at varying levels of efficiency in different individuals. This leads to some conception of an optimal level of functioning. A deviation from this optimum is thus considered to be, in varying degrees, a malfunction or failure of the human mechanism. Disease is conceived as such malfunctioning of the system. Thus, F.C. Redlich of Yale University says that "the most important concern of medicine is the cure and prevention of disease."[1] Health, in any other sense than the mere absence of disease, lies outside the purview of medicine as Redlich conceives it. One medical authority, W.R. Barclay, supports this view by emphatically distinguishing medical care from health care. Speaking of the correct uses of medical services in a community, Barclay says that "health care is not synonymous with medical care. Measurements that supposedly reflect health such as morbidity, longevity, growth and development are not measures of the quality of medical care being received."[2]

Causes of Disease

Medicine generally regards disease as an irregularity, a disorder, or a malfunction. This implies that at least ideally the human body can exhibit total regularity, orderliness, and flawless functioning. Of course, there are a great variety and a very great number of circumstances in which this orderliness and regularity can be interrupted, leading to the disorder we call disease. Nevertheless, there seem to be only three ways by which such deranging circumstances can come into being: (1) failure of homeostasis,[3] (2) heredity, and (3) intrusion of foreign substances (e.g., microbes, viruses, chemicals). Obviously, these three channels are not necessarily vehicles of disease only. Evidently the ingestion of substances or the inheritance of certain traits is part of the "normal" life of the body. Even such failures of homeostasis as occur in fever may not themselves be regarded as causes of disease. Quite the contrary, the production of fever may be a benign curative reaction to some disease.

These are not mutually exclusive channels of derangement, for it is conceivable for some pattern in failure of the regulatory mechanism to be due to hereditary influences. It is also possible that a failure of homeostasis is what made the body susceptible to infection caused by the intrusion of some virus. In other words, in some specific malfunction or disease more than one of these ways may be involved. Nevertheless, it is important to recognize the distinct characteristics of these three ways.

Failure of Homeostasis

Claude Bernard developed the idea that it is useful to think of the cells as existing in an internal environment, what he called the *milieu interieur*.[4] Every organism lives by interacting with its external environment. The body cells and fluids operate in much the same way in relation to their environment. They exist because of the nature of the interaction between their external environment and themselves.

The human body is a vast complex system of processes: blood circulates, the heart pumps, cells carry on various metabolic activities, heat is generated, tissues are nourished. There are many variations within these processes: temperature increases or decreases, as does blood pressure, pulse, respiration. The circulation varies in velocity; the diameter of blood vessels changes as does the viscosity of the blood.

One of the primary goals of the system is self-preservation. (Other goals include growth and reproduction.) There exists in living bodies a mechanism, a regulatory subsystem that maintains a constant internal environment within certain limits. The cells are bathed in fluids that act as intermediaries with the external environment. The external environment is continually changing the properties of the fluids, such as the blood, within specific limits, but the body's regulatory mechanisms counteract these external influences in such a way that a constant cellular environment is maintained. Bernard stated that "a higher organism is so constructed that if its dynamic equilibrium is slightly upset in one direction, reactions take place which tend to restore the balance."[5] The reactions are due to the regulatory mechanisms within the body. For example, in order to maintain the body temperature at about 37° C, the operation of several physiologic mechanisms is required. Loss of body heat results in vasoconstriction of surface vessels and erection of bodily hair. Adrenalin discharge then accelerates combustion, producing more heat in the body, and shivering increases heat because it is a form of muscular exercise.

Norbert Wiener points out that the condition of homeostasis is not limited to just the so-called vital functions, such as temperature control, cardiac function, respiration, and enzyme activity. It even extends to those functions that, if absent, are not considered life threatening, like the maintenance of posture and gait. Our ability to stand erect is due to negative feedback mechanisms, that is, those events that bring on a reaction in the opposite direction and thus cancel an original error in performance. "One's equilibrium in posture is the result of a continuous tendency to fall over in a direction opposite to that in which one has been previously falling. While standing and beginning to fall forward, the kinesthetic sensation produced by the stretching of the calf muscles starts a reflex which contracts them and pulls the person erect."[6] Such regulatory mechanisms within the body remain operative only within narrow limits. Should some external cause force the body beyond such limits, the homeostatic system breaks down and cannot supply compensatory adjustment without external assistance. For example, extreme cold in the environment might cause the body temperature to drop to an extremely low level (freezing) from which the body cannot recover. These limits of variation of the body's functioning define the healthy state. Thus, all vital functions undergo variation. When these variations exceed the normal limits, the body begins to show indications or malfunction or disorder and the need for external assistance. The health of the body consists of that state in which the proper functioning of the regulatory mechanism is maintained. Failure of the regulatory mechanism is the occasion for the intervention of the physician.

Bernard's ideas concerning physiologic functioning have been continually extended during the past hundred years, resulting in the development of the concept of organization, now used in contemporary physiology. One characteristic of physico-chemical systems is organization. The organism is viewed as being comprised of many physiologic subsystems operating at different levels of organization. The levels of organization reflect the degree of complexity of the functions the system serves. The philosopher Stephen Toulmin has described it as:

> The localized functions of individual organs and systems are interrelated. The larger scale systems perform more complex functions. The system integrity and regular operation of the constituent smaller scale systems would then be a precondition for healthy outcomes from the larger scale systems they make up.[7]

This provides a more general and more abstract conception of health. Without specifying the various subsystems of which the total organism is composed, health is seen as the integrity and effective interaction of the subsystems.

Heredity

We know that certain diseases can be traced to causes occurring prior to birth. There are two types of such prenatal causes. One type occurs in the uterine environment of the gestating individual; the other occurs in the genes of the parental reproductive cells. The latter type is termed the genetic cause of disease.

Inheritance of traits does not necessarily mean a resemblance between offspring and parent with respect to some trait, for inheritance may not be directly from the parents but through the parents from some earlier ancestor.

Disease is a heritable trait since it comes through the reproductive system. The treatment and cure of the disease is not precluded by the fact that it was transmitted through the reproductive cells. Nothing in the nature of inheritance precludes the possibility of a cure being discovered, although there are many such congenital diseases for which we do not now have a cure.

Medical scientists started studying the principles of heredity when it became clear that the study of the chemical nature of the genes could help in understanding the ways in which genes contribute to the growth and development of the body. It has been shown that certain genetic conditions can result in abnormalities in bodily structure and function. Scientists are thus studying the mechanisms responsible for the inheritance of anemias such as sickle-cell disease; searching for the etiologies, signs, and symptoms of inborn metabolic errors like phenylketonuria, and the genetic factors that influence the occurrence of chromosomal aberrations such as Down's syndrome.

Intrusion of Foreign Substances

Foreign substances that can cause malfunction or disease in the body are of two types, microbial and chemical. Usually, large numbers of microbes are active in the causation of disease. These large numbers may be engendered in the body in two ways. Some microbes enter the susceptible body and multiply or a large number of microbes enter the susceptible body from outside. Chemical substances can cause malfunction when they are inhaled, ingested, absorbed, applied to the body, or injected into it.

The disorder created by the action of microbes and chemicals in cells and tissues results in tissue injury or destruction. Physiologic response to these substances constitutes the inflammatory process— temperature rise, redness, swelling, antibody formation—detectable by the tools available to the medical doctor.

Concepts of Normal

Underlying these three concepts of physiology is the notion that there are pathophysiologic changes that can be identified by the medical doctor as transgressions from the normal. The idea that through the process of diagnosis a physician can identify various organic aberrations presupposes the existence of a norm—a standard from which the organism may be regarded as deviating. What then is this norm? In this discussion, two concepts of the normal will be considered: the normal as a statistical central tendency, and the normal as the ideal.

The Statistical Norm

This concept of the normal is identified with measurements typical of a population. The normal in this case is based on actual observation and is identified with the average. The average shows a characteristic of the collection of observations made; it shows the tendency of the variation in the collection. The tendency of the data to go in a certain direction is the central tendency and is given in one of these concepts: mean, median, mode. The normal in this statistical situation is taken as the central tendency.

Why should we regard the central tendency as normal? Since averages are derived from the study of actual cases, there can be certain advantages to the use of the term in this sense. In medical practice, the statistical normal is determined by calculating the central tendency of some measurable characteristic within a selected population. Thus, such useful norms as usual organ size, blood values, urine values, and blood pressure are obtained in this way.

Since this conception of the normal is based on actual observed conditions, the application of such a norm to an individual signifies that the aim of treatment is to bring the individual into conformity with the conditions typical of the actual population. The individual is not expected to improve beyond this, as contrasted with the ideal. Conformity is enough.

The Normal as the Ideal

The *optimal* level of functioning of the physico-chemical system is the normal function. Normal within this context is defined as "that which functions in accordance with its design."[8] The ideal physiologic system is not derived from studies of actual populations but from studies of general physiology. The function of an organ or a system implies its optimum or ideal level of operation. Once we know the physiologic function of the lungs within the human body, then by implication we have established the ideal level of performance of the lungs. This ideal level is the level of optimum efficiency. A system in which all elements perform their functions at an optimal level is the ideal system. In other words, the ideal is derived from the knowledge of function. For example, if the function of the lungs is to pass oxygen from the air into the blood and carbon dioxide from the blood into the air, then lung tissue needs to be elastic, with a rich blood supply, and have no obstruction to air or blood flow.

Once it is known that the heart is a pump, then its optimal operations can be inferred. The tissues and muscles of the heart must be strong enough to send blood all over the body. The valves within the heart must close at certain times. For example, the intake valve must be fully closed when the pump is expelling fluid or else there is a backflow. The pressure needed in the pump is determined by resistance to flow within the pipes, which must be kept clear of all obstructions in order to decrease resistance to flow. Thus, the notion of function is an empirical concept, based on actual physiologic characteristics of the body.

The norm as ideal is not a speculative subject but is based on the empirical science of physiology. The norm as ideal is not confined to actual populations. It gives one the vantage point of criticism of a population. This makes it possible to say that "A" has too much plaque in his vessels that interferes with optimal cardiovascular function. A statistical norm can only say what is typical of a population. The ideal norm provides a basis for setting up goals for improvements in the general conditions of mankind. One can also get an idea of what constitutes the ideal by knowing what pathology in an organ system is. The opposite of pathology would be the ideal.

Since medicine is based primarily on the conception of man as a physico-chemical system, the physician needs a grasp of the theoretical principles underlying this notion. Hence, doctors study the theories and methods of specific natural sciences (physics, chemistry) and the biological sciences (anatomy, physiology, microbiology) in order to guide their practices. Physicians must understand the human cardiovascular system in order to deal with a patient's heart problem. Insofar as physicians try to intervene in the behavior of patients in an effort to change unhealthy life styles, they will also need to be familiar with the theories of the behavioral sciences. The study of these sciences familiarizes them with what constitutes the ranges of normal and abnormal for these fields of study. Human beings thus present diverse aspects according to the scientific perspective from which they are viewed. They are mechanisms from the point of view of anatomy and physiology, organisms from the point of view of interaction with the environment, behavioral systems from the viewpoint of the behavioral sciences. In each of these areas, medicine is interested not only in describing a person from these viewpoints but also in defining normal status. It is in relation to such conceptions of the optimum or normal that medicine identifies diseases and illnesses.

Medicine as technique focuses on clinical experience. Armed with the understanding of general principles and faced with a patient, physicians try to associate clinical findings with underlying physiologic and pathophysiologic mechanisms. They attempt to identify the ranges of normal and abnormal in a specific human organism through the tools of practice, which include:

1. The medical history, which is the "chronicle of an individual life considered and digested with selective attention to the episodes significant for current diagnosis and treatment."[9]
2. The physical examination, performed in order to compare a specific person's constitution, conduct, appearance, subsystem functioning (using the techniques of observation, percussion, palpation, auscultation) with the standards of normal established by means of experiment and clinical experience.
3. Use of x-rays and laboratoɪy analysis of bodily fluids, secretions, and excretions in order to determine physiologic and biochemical functioning more precisely.

These tools of practice are used routinely to establish a baseline for judging future examination results and to uncover abnormalities.

By taking a history from a patient and performing a physical examination and laboratory tests, there are two types of information obtained. One type is couched in egocentric statements, such as, "I have heartburn." Asking, "Where is the pain?" and "How long does it last?" leads to egocentric responses. Physicians must depend on such egocentric statements because they have no objective way of obtaining such information except by asking the patient. The second type of information obtained is of an objective historical nature: "Have you seen any other physicians? Did you have this trouble before; where were you treated?" In asking these types of questions, physicians do not necessarily have to count on the patient for the information. They can get it from other sources such as past records and other physicians, but if the patient is a reliable historian, asking is faster. If the patient is not a reliable historian, the physician can ask other people, like a relative. In the case of a very young child, the physician would ask for such historical information from the parents. In performing a physical examination and interpreting laboratory tests, physicans are collecting objective data. They are making certain determinations based on what is seen, heard, felt, or smelled. They do not ask their patients for their blood pressure or rate of pulse or respiration because the state of physiology has advanced to the point where these kinds of determinations can be made independently of the patient's statements.

It would seem that physicians, because of their grasp of general scientific principles and the integration of this understanding with their clinical experiences, have a solid foundation upon which to make sound judgments about a particular patient's health status. However, except for instances of "classical textbook" disease conditions in patients, this is not so. This scientific knowledge, combined with an understanding of the uniqueness of each individual, will provide the physician with only "more or less articulate; more or less intuitive"[10] evidence upon which to base a diagnosis of sickness or health. The nature of diagnosis and prognosis is tentative and highly individualized because of an "intrinsic uncertainty about all particular applications of general scientific principles"[11] in practice and the consequences for individual patients. Knowing the general principles of cardiac function is one thing; understanding the specifics of Joe's heart is another matter.

Human psychology and physiology are very complex subjects, and our knowledge of the material is sparse. There is a great deal that we do not know about the human organism: what causes the heart to beat, the nature of fever, the cause of the feeling of hunger, the function of the brain, and so on.

Even when a diagnosis of disease is made, the disease process may not be clearly understood. The etiology of the condition may not be known. In this case, treatment is geared toward reducing or eliminating signs and symptoms. In many cases of disease, adequate treatment may not be available, or may not be known. If treatment is available, the patient may refuse it because of personal or financial considerations.

The nature of individuality is hidden in darkness.[12] We know that each person is different from every other person in morphological, psychological, and physiological characteristics. We also know that both heredity and environment contribute to nearly every human trait. What we do not know is how far a specific individual deviates from the general principles and experiences upon which medical practice is based.

Regardless of such uncertainties, physicians in the clinical situation are faced with the task of making decisions about the health status of their patients. This is, after all, their job. In order to make such decisions, physicians must have a working definition of normal. This working definition is based, in part, on the general principles of the relevant sciences. But the determination of a state of health or disease in practice involves more than this. The patient has to be viewed in relation to a standard of health.

Statements in general are either descriptive or evaluational. A norm or standard may be both descriptive and evaluational. A statement outlining the qualities constituting the norm is a descriptive statement, such as, "This is a book." But when that norm is used as a means of appraisal, as in, "This book is a *good* book," it becomes evaluational. An evaluative statement expresses some kind of preference or choice, whereas a descriptive statement is neutral with respect to preference.

The idea of norm is more general than the idea of value. Therefore, value is a kind of norm that expresses desire. Driving on the right side of the road is a norm in some societies. There has been an agreement to do it. We could decide to drive on the left side instead. The point is that there is no human desire involved here, so this standard is not a value.

Health, within this context, is a normative term. It constitutes a standard by which physicians can judge the physico-chemical condition of each person. But health can be viewed not only as normative but evaluational. When the state of health is equivalent to a condition of man regarded as the ideal state, that is, as a desirable and admirable state, health in this sense is a value expressing some kind of preference or choice. Disease is also a normative term but when used with health as an ideal state, disease within this context is also evaluational.

There may be some merit in distinguishing disease from illness. Such distinction may have a bearing in cases when an individual, despite a diseased condition of the body, presents a cheerful, optimistic aspect and carries on normal social and vocational functions. For the analysis of such cases it may be useful to consider "health" and "illness" as referring to the psychological attitude and behavioral patterns of an individual while "disease" and "the absence of disease" refer to the anatomical or physiological conditions of the body. We may thus speak of a person whose body "suffers" from some disease, but who is nevertheless not ill in the foregoing sense. On the other hand, we could describe a person as ill because of some detrimental qualities in his attitude and deficiencies in behavior even though there is no trace of disease in his body. These distinctions may have some special use in the consideration of the role-performance model of health. Thus, a person adequately performing his role would be considered well or healthy despite some ailment a physician can detect in his body.

What then is a disease and what is its relationship to illness? Are they equivalent terms? Feinstein defines the term disease in a manner which indicates that illness is not exactly identical with disease. He defines disease as "a condition which has a taxonomic vocabulary making description possible in the objective terminology of morphology, chemistry, microbiology, and physiology."[13] Objective changes in the mechanisms underlying normal physiological conditions of the body result in the pathophysiologic condition of disease. A viral infection of the body with the concomitant morphologic and biochemical bodily changes is a condition of disease. Calling this condition an illness introduces a new element into the discourse. The concept of illness involves a relationship between the diseased body and some antecedently conceived standard or normal condition of the body. In addition to the disease, it refers to an evaluation of the disease condition on the scale of the health-illness continuum. It is important to recognize that the identification of signs and symptoms of disease involves only descriptive phrases or statements. The term "illness" is evaluational. The physician who calls a patient ill goes beyond the mere fact of disease. That physician is formulating an evaluative statement on the basis of the evidence: signs, symptoms, test results, and so on. This evaluation is made by comparison with some norm. A person is called ill because he deviates from the standard of what a person's health should be. A disease of the body has so altered his condition and status that as compared with an optimal condition or optimal behavior pattern this person falls short.

He deviates from the ideal; he is ill. This is an evaluational statement.

While disease is a condition that can be described, illness is something more than that. It presents a situation that can be evaluated. It is possible to have two people, both with bronchitis. Both have a condition that shows pathology, but one may be more ill than the other. This evaluation is based on observation of characteristics of the two people other than just the presence of a disease condition. A top athlete will respond differently to the infection than a sedentary, malnourished individual. A football player who has a cold but does everything he is supposed to do in a game—score touchdowns, and so on—can be viewed as having a disease that he has evaluated as a low level illness. Of course, this situation raises questions about the wisdom of such a player. It is possible that without taking certain precautions the disease could become progressive. If he continues to disregard his disease, he could deteriorate, develop complications like pneumonia, and die. One might then say paradoxically that he died not of his illness but of his disease.

On the other hand, the term illness may refer not to a pathological condition of the body but to a mental or personality disorder or a behavioral aberration. Characterizing these disorders and aberrations as "illness" signifies their evaluation on the health-illness continuum scale.

The descriptive and evaluative terms used in medicine are not always obvious. The idea of disease being present in the body is descriptive. It states a verifiable fact—verifiable by normal medical judgment. One thinks of a disease as an objective condition manifesting certain observable characteristics. A condition of disease can produce certain signs that indicate an abnormality somewhere in the body. The signs are objective in that they are not dependent upon the patient's report; that is, they can be recognized by observation and physical examination by someone other than the patient. (Signs include such things as heart murmurs, jaundice, limping, and so on.) To say that someone is diseased refers implicitly to some preexisting syndrome or observed condition. For example, to say that a person has cholera signifies implicitly that the person has a temperature of 105°, diarrhea, dehydration, and coliform bacilli in his stool. The report of these signs is part of the objective description of the disease.

Disease also entails symptoms that are observable only by the patient. The physician can make only indirect observations of symptoms such as pain, headache, chills, or feelings of distress. For the awareness of these symptoms, the physician must depend on reports by the patient. The statements the patient formulates in reporting the subjective perceptions of the symptoms have a distinctive logical character. They are egocentric statements; that is to say, they are statements verifiable only by the speaker. For example, the patient's report: "I now feel a pain in my left shoulder," can be verified only by the patient at the present state of our knowledge of such psychophysiological phenomena.

Egocentric statements, in other words, are subjective. Whether there are always equivalent objective statements remains to be investigated. To put the problem more precisely consider the following assertions:

> *Jones:* I now feel a pain in my left shoulder.
> *Physician:* Jones feels a pain in his left shoulder.

The question raised here is the following: Is it possible to find confirming evidence of the latter statement other than the former?

Medical diagnosis may not reveal any symptoms or signs of derangement in people, but nothing can be inferred concerning their vigor, vitality, zest, stamina, or capacity to perform their accustomed roles. In this respect the functioning of the human body is analogous to the operation of a complex machine. The effectiveness or efficiency of the machine may vary over a wide range. There may be a great difference between the condition of the machine in which it and its several parts are merely functioning without derangement and the condition in which it functions at optimum effectiveness.

Is the optimization of the body-mind system as viewed within this context within the scope of medical practice? Or does the concern of medicine stop with the elimination of disease? Perhaps further improvement toward an optimum condition entails considerations that transcend medicine, and have to do with a way of life. In the final analysis, health may be a moral and political problem as much as it is a medical one.

Conclusion

Within the context of the clinical model, health has been defined as the absence of disease. This definition of health has been largely the result of the domination of the biomedical sciences by a mechanistic conception of man. Man is viewed by physicians primarily as a physico-chemical system.

Medical science views disease as a derangement, malfunction, or disorder that seems to result from a failure of homeostasis, hereditary error, or intrusion by foreign substances. The pathophysiologic changes resulting from the aforementioned processes can be diagnosed by medical doctors as deviations from a standard of normal—specifically, from a statistical norm or from an optimal level of functioning. In the former, the measurements are based on actual populations, and the use of this norm encourages conformity to the usual. In the latter instance, the norm as ideal encourages the use of standards that would improve one's general health.

The analysis in the foregoing chapter makes an implicit reference to two distinct perspectives of human nature. From one point of view, man is a machine—a complex, mechanical-physiologic system. From another point of view, man is a social-psychological person. Disease is a category that pertains to the former perspective; illness pertains to the latter. The idea of illness entails evaluation, whereas the idea of disease is confined to description. This makes it possible to place a disease condition on the scale of the health-illness continuum. Just as it is possible using the continuum to say that some people are healthier than others, so too is it possible to say that some people differ in degrees of illness.

Chapter 6

ROLE-PERFORMANCE MODEL

A role is a social norm or expectation of behavior. A person assuming a role undertakes to behave in conformity to these norms and to assume the duties and responsibilities entailed in them. The ability to conform to these norms and expectations is, from the viewpoint adopted here, a mark of health. Conversely, to the degree that individuals assuming roles lack the ability to perform at the expected level, they are, to that degree, ill.

Sickness then, within this context, is the kind of incapacity that prevents persons from "doing their jobs." If nothing in their condition impedes the effective performance of their roles, then they are, according to this view, in a healthy condition.

Several leading sociologists tend to view health as a social concept. Within this sociological context, where the individual is seen as part of a larger society, the healthy person is one who performs his or her preeminent roles. Because a person fulfills many roles—such as friend, parent, teacher, consumer, runner—the central or preeminent roles are those associated with one's family life and occupation.

Talcott Parsons, the well-known social theorist, says that:

it would be well to attempt to state . . . what seem to be the principle general characteristics of health and illness seen in the context of social role structure and social control. Health may be defined as the state of optimum capacity of an individual for the effective performance of the roles and tasks for which he has been socialized. It is defined with reference to the individual's participation in the social system and also relative to his status in society.[1]

Twaddle concurs. "From the social standpoint, perfect health may be a state in which an individual's capacities for task and role-performance are optimized."[2] Robert Wilson adds, "Normal health consists of the ability to perform adequately in the individual's chief social roles, notably the familial and the occupational. . . ."[3]

With this social perspective of health and disease in mind, David Mechanic, a leading medical sociologist, states that the onset of disease and illness "may depend not only upon the personal characteristics of people but also upon the degree of fit between the person and the social position he assumes or is thrust upon him."[4] In other words, how well people are qualified to do what they have taken on or what they are forced to do may determine their state of health. It is conceivable that a very active person, such as an explorer, who earns his living by mapping unknown lands and thrives in the out-of-doors life would become ill if he suddenly had to lead the life of an office manager.

While all these spokesmen identify health as role-performance, there are differences of formulation and emphasis among them. For Wilson, health is that condition in which an individual is able to perform his role satisfactorily. It is important to note that the criterion of health in this context is not the actual performance of the role but the ability for such performance. There are, of course, degrees of performance. Correspondingly, there are degrees of health. As Twaddle says, "Perfect health may be a state in which an individual's capabilities for role and task performance are optimized."[5] The capacity for performance may exist even when the individual abstains from or refuses such performance. As Parsons notes in his writing, he is not referring to the successful fulfillment of specific types of roles.[6] Whether a man actually assumes responsibility for the care of his children is not the issue. A man can choose not to nurture his family, but nevertheless would still be considered healthy in this sociological context as long as his abilities and capacities to fulfill such responsibilities are intact.

The ability of the individual to meet the demands created by various roles helps determine his or her degree of health. Most people are able to perform at some acceptable level in their chief social roles. It seems that few people are able to function equally well in all their social roles. Most people, who may not be able to perform adequately in one particular kind of role, have the capabilities to perform adequately in roles with other kinds of responsibilities. Take, for example, an individual who is a bookkeeper, parent, member of an amateur baseball team, and a member of the P.T.A. He may conceivably function as a very able bookkeeper but be far below the optimum in his role as husband and baseball player. In thinking of health in terms of role-performance, the focus is as noted above on some central preeminent role and, specifically, on the ability of the individual to perform his role. In the example above, he may in fact be a bad husband not because he lacks the ability to be a good one but because he is distracted by other amatory interests. He may be a bad baseball player not because he could not be a good one, if he put his mind to it, but because he is bored by the game. In other words, his being below optimum in these roles does not indicate a lack of *ability* to perform and, consequently, does not indicate a failure of health.

According to Parsons, what this criterion signifies is that health is the condition in which the person has the ability to perform his role, even though he may not necessarily be performing it. But how does one know when a person has the ability? The determination of this ability can only be made by observing the actual performance. In other words, the best way to determine if A has the ability to perform task B is to ask A to perform it. The best criterion to determine fulfillment of a role is the performance of the role. In the final analysis, the criterion is in fact the actual performance of a role.

Another significant point to note concerning this role-performance criterion of health is that it is a variable criterion. It varies in relation to the social role and status to which it is applied.[7] Each kind of role makes its unique demands on the intellectual and personal equipment of the individual. The role of a writer demands different things than that of a laborer. Whereas the writer can lead a sedentary existence and still perform his job, physical stamina is one of the fundamental ingredients in the ability of the laborer to do his job. While the writer might be unable to detect even a significant decrease in the amount of his physical stamina, the laborer would be able to detect even a slight decrease in his. This notion is in contrast to that of the ideal man where a fixed set of qualities could be set forth that would serve to identify such a person.

The idea of health as role-performance is not limited to the experts. Adequate role-performance appears to be a "natural" commonsense criterion of health and a number of people as reported in medical sociology think of illness and health on this model. DiCicco and Apple, in studying a group of people 65 and over from the Roxbury district in Boston, found that the majority of their sample considered themselves healthy if they could maintain their usual activities of daily living—doing what had to be done, getting out of the house, being independent. This was also true among those who had minor ailments.[8]

Koos and his associates visited 500 families in an upper New York state town in an attempt to learn, among other things, their attitudes toward health and illness. The importance of an individual's role within the family was a factor in seeking medical care if that person was thought to be sick. One woman summarized this by stating, "If something were wrong with my husband, we'd get it fixed right away. He earns the money and we can't have him stop work."[9]

Suchman, utilizing information received from 137 respondents selected from the Washington Heights section of New York City who were part of another study, reports that "the more severe the individual's symptoms . . . and the more they interfere with his ability to carry on his usual activities, the more likely it is that he will think of himself as ill."[10]

Michael Grossman, an economist, has shown that a person's self-rating of his own health status—excellent, fair, good, or poor—is significantly correlated to the number of symptoms reported, time lost from work because of sickness, and medical expenses.[11]

In one sense, it is easy to understand how people would come to form the idea of health as role-performance. It is a commonsense notion derived from experience. Health has always had a component of function or performance. The incapacity or inability to perform one's usual functions, especially those associated with job and family, have generally led people to the idea that something was wrong, that is, they thought of themselves as sick.

The idea of role-performance can be said to have certain characteristics, such as efficiency (some people are more adequate than others in fulfilling their responsibilities), and endurance (the ability to perform over a long period of time). The term "role-performance" consequently signifies the ability to perform a role effectively over an adequate period of time. In other words, role-performance means effectiveness in one's role.

Thus, when psychologic or physiologic problems, such as depression or tremors, appear in a person, they are viewed as causing failures in the ability to efficiently perform one's role, like a job, over long periods of time. Even though the person may still appear to be carrying out his job, an astute observer such as an industrial engineer could see that he is not fulfilling his responsibilities efficiently or enduring them for a sufficient period. Although the individual in this condition may still continue in this role, the feeling of discomfort or distress associated with these problems may lead to undue fatigue, and in time hamper efficiency—resulting perhaps in eventual breakdown. In other words, if health is role-performance, a failure of health, that is, illness, may occur before a complete breakdown in performance. Loss of efficiency or undue fatigue are themselves signs of illness. They are objective counterparts of subjective symptoms like discomfort, distress, or pain.

Although usually the person feels well, the condition of subjective well-being is not regarded as an essential component of health conceived as role-performance. One can possibly do some jobs well even while experiencing subjective feelings of pain and distress. Under certain conditions, these feelings of distress or pain would be viewed as symptoms of some ailment requiring some degree of care. However, in performing some important role these distractions of discomfort and distress may very well be ignored. The extent to which the individual persists in the performance of a role despite such subjective symptoms will depend on motivation, interest, and economic dependence on the role. There is thus a certain ambiguity with regard to health status. A person is not well in light of the pain and distress but is well enough to perform a role with optimum effectiveness. That person is both well and ill, depending on whether the condition is appraised subjectively or in terms of objective performance.

Generally, the idea of health as role-performance occurs in association with other ideas about health, like health as freedom from signs and symptoms of disease. It appears that a person is able to distinguish between the subjective feelings of pain and distress and the necessity he may feel to still fulfill role responsibilities. Thus, while a person may accomplish the same amount of work when feeling ill as he does when feeling well, he can still recognize the subjective discomfort under which he continues to meet the demands of his various roles.

In characterizing health as role-performance, one cannot altogether exclude other conceptions, specifically, a clinical view of health. The distress and pain that the individual feels may, after all, be symptoms of a developing condition that may soon undermine the ability to perform. Clinically, he has an incipient illness or disease even while he may be regarded as a healthy performer in his role.

Within this context, disease can be seen in two aspects: static and dynamic. The static view conceives of disease as a syndrome of signs and symptoms regarded as qualities or conditions of the body, including blood glucose levels, blood pressure, and so on. From the dynamic viewpoint, disease is seen as a function of behavior. There are patterns of behavior that are characteristic of health and other patterns that are marks of illness. The idea of behavior involves activity, motion, exertion. Within this context health is efficiency, creativity, eptness, effectiveness. Illness is ineptness, inefficiency, ineffectiveness. The concept of health as role-performance belongs to this second category—the dynamic or behavioral idea of health.

Under some conditions behavior may appear to be random. But socialized behavior, that is to say, the behavior of socialized man, is organized into patterns with specific orientation toward social objectives. These patterns of behavior define the manner in which the individual participates in the structure and enterprises of the society of which he is a member. In other words, they define his role in the community.

A role is an essential part of the social structure and reflects the traditions of a society. It marks the most significant aspects of the relations into which an individual enters as a member of society. Within this sociological frame of reference, the term role refers to a part a person plays in society. The term is used in the same sense as it is used in the theater: individuals perform their roles as actors play their parts.[12] The actors, in both the sociological and theatrical senses of the word, learn a part and are expected to exhibit the behaviors, characteristics, and mannerisms called for by society in the one situation and by the playwright in the other. The actress assigned to play the part of a loving mother is expected to show the same personal traits and behavioral patterns as a woman who is, in fact, a loving mother.

Effective performance of our roles in society provides the foundation upon which our social institutions are built.[13] Social institutions such as the family, the schools, and the churches are composed of individuals who engage in a series of characteristic actions or behavior patterns. These behavior patterns are their roles. Such behaviors by individuals help determine the quality of the entire society. In other words, in order for our social institutions to perform their functions well, the individuals who make up these institutions must effectively fulfill the kinds of roles that ensure the maintenance of these institutions. For example, one role of the family is to nurture and educate the helpless young. This job must be done adequately in order for society as we know it to continue.

The development of role expectations has helped to ensure effective role-performance.[14] They are the means for evaluation of role-performance by the person assuming the role and by society in general. But in order to know what is expected when a role is assumed, the person who is to fulfill it must have the opportunity to learn what these behaviors are. When the person receives this information, he is then able to more effectively fulfill the requirements associated with the role. The orientation period for new staff nurses in a hospital or clinic is an example of the methods used to assist people in learning what their behaviors should be.

Persons who assume the various roles of life are expected to conform to the usual standards of performance for these roles. When persons are viewed as adhering to the norms, their actions are considered legitimate. Consequently, they are likely to be effective in the performance of their roles. From time to time, issues are raised concerning a nurse's treatment of a patient. The question of legitimacy of the nurse's conduct is related to the idea of the nursing role. If the behavior follows from or is in accord with the accepted role of the nurse, then such conduct is legitimate. "Almost any form of behavior is acceptable . . . if it results from a role in society that is recognized as legitimate."[15]

The person who assumes a role is not viewed as being a passive recipient of these role expectations but as actively shaping, modifying, and adjusting the many different roles that will be assumed in a life. Thus, role behaviors are modified by both the individuals assuming them and by the continually changing social environment. New sets of roles are constantly evolving and other roles become obsolete as the social environment and individuals change. The birth of computer technology introduced previously unknown roles into our society: systems engineer, keypunch operator, programmer. With the rise of industrialization and science, other roles were less useful and declined, like that of cowboy, linotype setter, and medicine man.

Failure in Role-Performance

The foregoing discussion has focused on the components within the idea of role that generally create order and a sense of permanence in society. But performance as a model of health is complicated by the emergence of role conflicts. Role conflict or strain is defined as an aspect of social interaction occurring at two levels: within the individual and among people.[16] It involves competition within the individual and among people for the same object and takes the form of difficulty in resolving conflicting duties among simultaneously filled roles. While such conflict is considered to be present in varying degrees with every role, the amount of conflict increases when norms and expectations associated with the role are not clear, and with the diversity and number of roles and aspirations held. No one holds only one role in life. We all hold many roles, but we do not necessarily perform all our roles equally well. In fact, effective performance in one role may preclude adequate performance in another. Does health as role-performance mean filling all the roles of any one individual or does it mean filling most of these roles? How does one determine which of these roles should be filled and which should not? Within the context of health as role-performance, what could constitute a healthy life? One answer would be the capacity to fulfill one's roles with a minimal amount of role conflict. The individual who can harmonize all roles into one harmonious whole is the healthy person.

Parsons says that illness "is most generally characterized by some imputed generalized disturbance of the capacity of the individual for normally expected tasks or role performance."[17] This appears to be too sweeping in its generalizations. There are, after all, deficiencies and disturbances that interfere with role-performance but would not be considered instances of illness or disease. In other words, while performance of one's role indicates health, failure in performance does not necessarily indicate illness. People may fail in role-performance for many reasons: they may lack the skills required in the role; they may be unsuitable for the role; they may be distracted by other prevailing interests; or they may be unwilling to assume the responsibilities entailed in the role. Any one of these circumstances may result in failure in role-performance.

It should also be noted that there are two different kinds of failures in role-performance. The first occurs when a person has the intention of succeeding, assumes the role, is willing to engage in it, but fails. The second kind of failure usually occurs when the role is foisted upon the individual, who then fails because of lack of interest or motivation. He fails because, despite his effort, he does not really want to succeed. Neither of these instances is necessarily indicative of illness. If a man, for example, is not skilled in his job or hates it, he would not be considered ill and would not need the services of a physician, but he might benefit from a vocational training program.

In speaking of failure in role-performance, it is of course assumed that in some way the individual was motivated to perform the role. There are distinct motives for assuming a role and a consideration of these motives is not irrelevant to the appraisal of failure or success in the role. The expectation of satisfaction, the fear of painful consequences, or a sense of duty may each serve as motives in role-performance. However, the individual may assume a role because of social tradition or habit, in other words, without conscious choice or evaluation. Whether the situation involves the former explicit motives or is confined to the implicit customs or constraints of tradition, the role invariably entails a certain socialization of the individual. The role itself is a form or criterion of such socialization. The individual is expected to conform to these criteria either by submission to the constraints of custom or by reflective choice among roles available to him. In this sense, socialization is a sine qua non of role-performance.

Under what conditions then does a failure in role-performance indicate illness? If a person *intends* to fulfill his role responsibilities and his past record indicates that he can, in fact, do so but on some occasion he fails in his performance, such failure may be regarded as a mark of illness. What are the specific conditions under which the failure in performance may justifiably be called illness or disease? The following suggest themselves as possible conditions of this kind.

1. The inability to meet the clinical requirements of health. The individual is not physiologically sound and manifests signs and symptoms of malfunction or derangement.
2. The individual is clinically sound but fails to meet the social requirements of the role. There are circumstances in which socialization of the individual in a role is never attained or where once attained it is weakened or disrupted. A variety of psychological conflicts and aberrations may result in such a social failure. A mind not at rest because of conditions in the immediate social environment, like family stress, can result in illness and disease. It is possible that the many roles a person willingly assumes do not blend harmoniously with his personality. He might not be able to adjust or adapt to the various role demands because he might be hampered by all kinds of anxieties and self-doubts. The degree of adjustment to such role demands could be inadequate, creating a sense of internal disharmony. This disharmony could lead to such behavioral disturbances as agitation, moodiness, short-temper—all indicative of a possible impending failure in role-performance. Thus, the aforementioned conditions could result in failures of role-performance indicating illness and disease. Such failures in role-performance have not generally been considered illness but within this context, they are.

Conclusion

In the foregoing, health is defined as the ability to fulfill one's central roles. A role is a sociological construct and refers to the pattern of organized behaviors people assume in society. The central roles are generally those associated with one's family responsibilities and occupation. Illness, within this context, is the inability to perform at expected levels in one's roles. Studies show the tendency of laymen to conform to this conception of illness. They see themselves as ill when they note their own failures in maintaining customary effectiveness in the performance of their roles. It is noted, on the other hand, that under some conditions persons continue in the effective performance of their roles despite the presence of clinically identifiable disease.

There are two kinds of failures in role-performance. The first occurs in situations where people may want to succeed but do not have the skills to do so. The second kind occurs when people lack interest or motivation in the role. Thus, while adequate role-performance indicates health within this context, failure in role-performance does not necessarily indicate illness.

The role-performance model provides a fairly minimal conception of health because it can be viewed as focusing only on the individual's social fitness. The ranges of human behaviors are broader. People may fall short of the clinical model in that they may be physiologically ill even though able to fulfill their central roles. People able to perform adequately in their occupational or familial roles may fail altogether to achieve the self-actualization of Maslow's model or the adaptive facility of Dubos's model, which will be discussed in the following chapters.

Chapter 7

ADAPTIVE MODEL

The adaptive idea of health developed in the writings of René Dubos, the eminent microbiologist and experimental pathologist, is based on a generalized conception of medicine that includes but extends beyond the study and treatment of diseases.[1] In this context, health is the condition of the whole person engaged in effective and fruitful interaction with the physical and social environment. The characteristic mode of this interaction is adaptation or adaptive behavior. Thus, disease is a failure in adaptation. It is a breakdown in the ability of the organism to cope with certain changes in its environment. Medical treatment aims to restore this ability so the organism can once again function by means of its own adaptive mechanisms.

According to this conception, even when individuals have been freed of disease, they may still not have attained health. They may still fail in effective functioning in the social scene. Privations of all kinds—food, wholesome air, recreation, education, and others—may confront them with hostile, challenging environments with which they cannot cope and to which they are unable to adapt. For Dubos, this condition also marks the absence of health.

Types of Adaptation

Health as viewed by Dubos refers to a life conducted in such a way that the individual adapts and adjusts to continually changing environmental conditions. Successful adaptation to varying environmental situations requires effective interactions with the environment. Adaptation is a characteristic of human life and Dubos distinguishes between two types: biological and social. Biological adaptation refers to successful responses to environmental challenges by an organism that develops the physico-chemical mechanisms to deal with them. Such environmental conditions change from one place to another and the organisms inhabiting those areas must successfully adapt to those changes in order to remain healthy. Eskimos can ride their dog sleds barechested in −30°F arctic weather and certain Australian aborigines can store water in their stomachs in order to endure desert conditions.[2] A New Yorker would never survive in either of these situations without the benefit of proper technological aids.

But, Dubos says, such biological adaptive ability is not limited to those developed over centuries by means of hereditary processes. Temporary adaptive mechanisms can be found in individuals who need to function in new environments. The vacationer from New York City who spends the summer running in the mountains surrounding Santa Fe, New Mexico will in a few weeks develop the increased respiratory depth and hemoglobin needed to train in that environment. The return to New York City will generally entail a return to the usual physiologic state, provided the person is healthy.

Biological adaptation is also expressed in behavior patterns—the instincts, tastes, and habits—that Dubos calls a type of biological learning. We exhibit broad ranges of behavior changes because we have learned from our past experiences. These kinds of learning patterns are transmitted to other individuals and groups. Dubos considers such diverse phenomena as acquired immunity and customs, taboos, and religious beliefs as results of biological learning and adaptive practices.

The adaptive faculties of the human being go far beyond biological capabilities. They are augmented by what Dubos calls conscious social processes. He says that our abilities to socially adapt "have been the most influential determinants of man's fate during historical times."[3] Man can, to a large extent, change "the physical world to suit his requirements."[4] It is with this point in mind that Dubos, in one of his public lectures, made the comment that man is no longer subject to evolutionary laws and, in a sense, this is true. He no longer needs to be subjected to the laws of natural selection because of the advances made in his technology. Prior to such technological development, the environment determined the conditions under which organisms had to adjust. A cold, wintry climate meant that the kinds of organisms that could survive there had thick, furry coats. A hot dry climate was kinder to those with dark pigmentation and very little body hair. An aquatic environment necessitated the development of some kind of gill system. But it is conceivable that man can meet any environmental change, not through organic evolution, but through technological skills. If the polar ice cap were to begin melting at a rate that would inundate massive tracts of land, it is conceivable that man, through science and technology, could build undersea communities in which to live, and develop the tools necessary to farm and utilize the resources of the ocean floor. Or he might choose to build a spaceship and go to another planet or live in a space station. In any case, he would be molding the environment to his needs. He would not have to significantly change himself in order to survive and grow.

However, the more effective attack on disease and more enduring fundamental cultivation of health rests in the way man and the environment interact. John Dewey, the twentieth-century American philosopher, discusses two aspects of adaptation. Adaptation, he says, is "quite as much adaptation of the environment to our activities as of our activities to the environment."[5] Thus, the adjustment of the organism to the environment results in the ability to change that environment. The changed environment then becomes the means to further modify the activities of the organism. One can imagine a community where poverty, disease, malnutrition exist. In such a community, two contrasting social outlooks might emerge. On the one hand, a type of conservative outlook would assert that these environmental conditions are tests that challenge the people who live there. Those who are tough enough can cope with the conditions, survive, and perhaps even flourish. They survive because they are superior. Others who are not so fortunate die or live a debilitating kind of existence. In this viewpoint, the demands are placed on the individual—adapt or die. This is the view of Social Darwinism, the extension of biological evolutionary thought into the study of society.[6] As Dewey notes, this kind of adaptation involves "a maximum of accepting, tolerating, putting up with things as they are, a maximum of passive acquiescence, and a minimum of active control."[7]

There is an alternative viewpoint. In this case, the social philosophy rests on a critique of that society. Such an outlook does not view the situation as inevitable. The individual is not asked to cope with poverty and disease. Instead, such conditions are to be altered or eliminated through political action, public education, and so on. Such a philosophy of reform proposes that the social environment be adapted to individual needs rather than conversely, adapting the individual to the environment. The environment, in short, is to be made more conducive to human life.

According to our constitutional philosophy, we have an inalienable right to the pursuit of happiness. Is happiness possible without health? It is true that people suffering from incurable disease may achieve a kind of joy and serenity that lifts them above the pain and suffering. But happiness must mean something more than such stoic transcendence of suffering. It must mean a kind of enduring fullness of life. While some pain and disappointment may be unavoidable, happiness means a condition in which there is a large residue of satisfaction. If, as Thomas Jefferson says, we have a right to pursue such happiness, then by implication we have a right to seek those social and physical conditions without which such enduring happiness is not possible. A beneficent, health-giving environment thus becomes not the privilege of the fortunate few or the wealthy, but the right of everyone.

In Dubos's work, the adaptive concept of health takes into account a fundamental fact of life and human nature: change. Nothing is fixed. Health is not a static, stable condition in which man is placed in a kind of happy coordination with the environment. There can be no such static adjustment because the environment is not fixed. It is in a condition of continual modification and transformation, as is man. Fitness within the environment is achieved only through continual adaptation, adjustment, and awareness of change—actions that demand new attitudes and postures in the individual. Health is a process of change and interaction between man and the environment, but it is possible to attain a kind of equilibrium between the two in much the same sense as chemical equilibrium is reached between two fluids on each side of a semipermeable membrane when diffusion equalizes their concentration. It is possible for man to be alert and aware so that he can adapt to changes or change the environment to suit him. This dynamic equilibrium between man and the environment is never permanent. There is always threat of a change and a demand for new adaptation—so health is never completely and finally achieved. To put it paradoxically, health is the capacity of the individual to meet the ever present threats to his health.

Dubos says that man believes that perfect health and happiness are his attainable prospects, yet the processes of everyday life are a contradiction to that dream of paradise. He writes of the ancient Greeks who believed in the existence of happy races who lived in inaccessible parts of the world, and of the Chinese who wrote of human beings living beyond a hundred years of age without becoming ill and decrepit.[8] Almost every culture in the world has shared in some portion of this myth. Most dreams of paradise are simplified longings and ideals that obscure the complexities of the delicate biological and psychosocial organism. No such simplified dreams of paradise could be reconciled with the interactions of this vastly complex human system and its even more intricate natural environment.

Life in paradise is a static existence. There organismic life flows happily on without change or conflict with internal or external forces. But in the natural scene there are always intrusions—physical, biological, and social—in the face of which survival is possible only through adaptation. Without such adaptation there is little hope for growth and fulfillment. Thus, according to Dubos, the purpose of adaptation is growth, expansion, and creation. He is not speaking merely of biological adaptation but the development of what he considers far more meaningful aspects of man's nature: his psychosocial and spiritual nature. It is through these aspects that the more interesting adjustments of the organism have been made. He stresses that life must be structured in a way that will allow man to "search for the fundamental satisfactions found only in nature, in human relationships, and in self-discovery."[9]

While Dubos would never deny the importance of the proper order and functioning of organic physico-chemical mechanisms, such mechanistic order is not enough for health in this context. "Solving problems of disease is not the same thing as creating health and happiness. This [larger] task demands a kind of wisdom and vision . . . which apprehends in all their complexities and subtleties the relationship between living things and their total environment."[10] The total environment for Dubos includes the physical and social world, and the individual's perceptual and conceptual world. Not only must people be healthy in the clinical sense, they must have the capacity for reflection, interpretation, analysis, and the willingness to seek adventure. In short, the creative use of the intellect and the skillful use of social abilities is what Dubos means by health. Failure to adapt to the environment results in illness and disease.

This adjustment to the environment is far more complex than first thought. For example, healthy individuals often do not become ill, and at times cannot do so, even when they purposely expose themselves to large numbers of disease-producing microorganisms. Dubos cites the examples of Pettenkofer in Germany in 1900 and Metchnikoff in France who, with several of their assistants, drank tumblersful of cultures taken from people who died of cholera. The result was nothing more than mild diarrhea for a few of the experimenters, even though enormous numbers of cholera vibrios were recovered from their stools. Dubos states that even a larger number of virulent microorganisms in the body rarely results in disease. It appears that some other factor in addition to the microorganisms must be present to produce disease.

Implicit in Dubos's work is the idea that the interaction between the individual and the environment should be effective and fruitful. What is effective and fruitful may be indicated by the formulation of some "aim" of organic life. In this connection the concept of growth as developed by Dewey, which is implicit in Dubos's writings, will be examined.

Dubos states that "the activities of man seem to have on the whole a direction upward and forward which tends to better his life physically, intellectually, and morally."[11] The cumulative movement toward future results is what Dewey means by growth.[12] Growth within this context goes beyond biological purpose and technological development. Rather, Dewey's idea of growth is concerned not only with biological development but with intellectual and social growth; a continuous expansion of horizons and vistas of experiences; in other words, with a search for varieties of activities and experiences with the result that new purposes and goals are formulated and achieved. Certainly, a necessary condition for such human growth is a nurturing, stimulating environment that will foster and promote a high order of biological and social evolution, rather than one that hinders or inhibits such activities. In other words, the environment helps determine the kinds of activities individuals will engage in.

Since man is an active participant in the process of living, "a continuous readjustment" to the demands of his internal and external worlds is necessary. Hence, the possibilities for further development exist—for becoming or doing something different, Dewey says, once the results of one's actions are analyzed. The idea of growth is not focused on passive, frightened, untrying individuals but those adventurous, creative people who ultimately advance social evolution. Dewey emphatically states that the purpose of growing is to retain the capacity for further growth.[13] It should be a continuous process.

The Responsibility of Medicine

With reference to Dubos's concept of health, it may be noted that there are two viewpoints on the primary responsibility of medicine. One view calls for emphasis on the maintenance and promotion of health; the other for treatment and, when possible, for cure of disease conditions. Since health, viewed as a normal healthy mind in a normal healthy body, has been thought of as the customary human state, it appears that most people in the various cultures that we know have taken this state of wellness for granted. That is, they have never made as great an effort in trying to exemplify the fundamental reasons for states of robust health as they have for determining causes of disease conditions. Thus, much knowledge and skill have been devoted to developing treatments and restorative measures for people who are injured or diseased. Caring for the sick has generally been the most important function of medicine.

Nevertheless, from the time of the Hippocratics of ancient Greece to the present, the proponents of health have been active. They have generally maintained that the healthy state of the organism is related to the conditions in the organism's environment. An organism, in order to remain healthy, must be surrounded by salubrious conditions: clean air, water, housing, nourishing food, a safe workplace. This thinking had impressive results in a time such as that of the Industrial Revolution when large numbers of people were attracted to the cities because of the job opportunities. When they were forced to live in crowded and squalid conditions, they became ill. Their social and health problems were so acute that reform movements started up quickly and continued in force until the second half of the nineteenth century. The reformers believed that disease could be controlled by bringing back to the people pure air, water, and generally clean surroundings. Their social philosophy was basically a "back-to-nature" theme and the results were very effective. The general health of the working classes improved.

With the development of the scientific method and its application in the biological sciences, the problems concerning diseases were reformulated and experimentation began in the laboratory. The specific etiology of disease was the result. Poisons and germs within the organism were causing diseases, and for every cause of disease there was a promise of a specific treatment and cure for it. This theory has been very effective in dealing with many physiologic derangements. The doctrine of specific etiology has held the central position in medicine. Certainly Pasteur and Koch initially, and many experimental scientists after them, have proved that disease is caused by the presence of virulent microorganisms in the body. These researchers made important, even revolutionary, contributions to the theory of disease. But some questions have been raised concerning the adequacy of this doctrine of specific etiology. To some investigators it appears that other factors must be considered before we can gain a full understanding of the nature of disease. Writing of these developments, René Dubos has observed that

> Pasteur and Koch did not deal with natural events but with experimental artifacts. . . . By the skillful selection of experimental systems, Pasteur, Koch, and their followers succeeded in minimizing in their tests the influence of factors that might have obscured the activity of the infectious agents they wanted to study. This experimental approach has been extremely effective for the discovery of agents of disease and for the study of some of their properties. But it has led by necessity to the neglect, and indeed has often delayed the recognition, of the many other factors that play a part in the causation of disease under conditions prevailing in the natural world, for example, the physiological status of the infected individual and the impact of the environment in which he lives.[14]

Even drugs, writes Dubos, are not the panacea for the ills of mankind.[15] They are at best stop-gap measures, good in the short term despite dangerous drawbacks like allergies and poisoning effects. Drugs may kill specific microbes in the body, but the existence of these microbes in the organism is not the fundamental problem when attempting to understand the nature of health and disease. The microbial world, in fact, is only one part of a very complex ecological system. The characteristics of the entire physical and social environments as they relate to the human organism must be grasped, Dubos says, in order to understand the nature of human health and disease.

For Dubos, the road to health lies in the capacity of man to recognize and correct the mismanagements of lifestyle. Drugs, for example, may control the symptoms of heart disease but proper diet, exercise, cessation of smoking, and a positive attitude, that is, the choices which each individual can institute, may prevent it.

Man cannot sweep away the concrete and return to "nature." Even if that were possible, we know that it would not lead to health. But we can make the best of this situation by using our intelligence creatively, and perhaps then we will achieve all we are capable of achieving.

Dubos's ideas concerning the relationship of man with his environment appear to be extensions of certain of the Hippocratic medical ideas. The Hippocratics knew there were signs and symptoms that indicated that people had diseases. They knew these diseases generally had specific courses to follow and that the etiology of these disease conditions was somehow connected with the physical environment. They also knew treatment of these disease conditions involved a change in the patient's lifestyle.[16]

Dubos argues that the fundamental causes of diseases can only be understood when the environment is taken into account. The environment for Dubos is not limited to the physical environment but includes the social environment as well as man's internal environment, including his perceptual and conceptual worlds.[17] For example, anginal pain cannot only be viewed as a malfunction of the coronary arteries; it is also a physiological symptom that must be viewed from a perspective beyond that of the physico-chemical if the organism is to be adequately treated. Such pain is a serious symptom of coronary artery disease and can generally be relieved by nitroglycerine, a vasodilating medicine. However, the treatment of the underlying condition may not come through drugs or triple coronary by-pass surgery but through a complete change in lifestyle. The individual with angina may have to alter the ways he deals with stressful situations and events. His temperament may have to be changed from a hard-driving, time-oriented one to one that is more relaxed and flexible. Eating habits may need to be altered and exercise has to be incorporated into the individual's life. Smoking should cease and heavily polluted surroundings should be avoided. In short, aspects of both the individual's internal and external environment would have to be changed in order to decrease damage to the heart and blood vessels.

Another example illustrating this point is the notorious history of pellagra. Pellagra was shown by Goldberger to be due to the absence of niacin in the diet. The entire syndrome of this disease disappears in the individual when that one vitamin is restored to the diet. In this sense, we can speak of the absence of niacin in the diet as the specific cause of the disease called pellagra. But the cause of the disease can also be viewed as social and economic in nature. The people who develop this disease follow a certain pattern. They are the poor and ignorant whose living comes from farming. Consequently, they have access to and can afford to eat only certain kinds of foods. Until the 1940s, citizens of the southern United States who developed pellagra existed on diets of biscuits, grits, syrup, cornmeal, and gravy. While this diet is deficient in many nutrients, it is very low in niacin. Hence, the condition of the environment can be viewed as producing the deficiency-disease, pellagra. In order to understand the nature of pellagra, we have to know the environmental circumstances in which it arises. It is not enough to know that organismic signs and symptoms of the disease are produced by the absence of a specific vitamin in the diet. One must understand the kind of social and physical environmental conditions that are conducive to the development of the disease because clues to disease prevention result. The prevention of pellagra occurred by means of social action and not by the administration of niacin through the medical care system. Pellagra was eliminated in this country because of the enrichment of cereals and breads with yeast initially; niacin, thiamin, iron, and riboflavin were then added routinely in the early 1940s.[18] In this sense the idea of the adaptive model of health appearing in Dubos's books is an important directive idea serving to unite the aims of preventive as well as therapeutic medicine.

Adaptation and Cybernetic Theory

At this point, it would be useful to discuss adaptive behavior as an entirely naturalistic phenomenon that can be investigated by the empirical sciences. Since adaptive behavior can also be viewed in terms of teleological cosmology, it raises questions of immanent purpose or purposeful regulation pertaining to some nonmaterial mind or spirit. Scientific and technological development have led to a naturalization of the idea of the human person so we no longer need the hypothesis of nonmaterial agencies or elements to account for purposeful adaptive behavior. This differentiation is important in establishing health within this context as a natural phenomenon, like disease.

Is the living being governed by something other than the laws of material nature? Is the living being something more than material? Can the phenomenon of adaptive behavior be fully accounted for in terms of the properties of matter and material structure? In other words, is adaptive behavior found only in living beings?

There are, of course, many characteristics of the living body that seem to distinguish it fundamentally from the nonliving. For example, if the human body is cut on its skin, it will marshall its physiologic resources in such a way that will result in the mending of the damage done by the trauma to the skin and underlying tissue. But if the cylinder head of an engine is cut, it will remain damaged. It has no way to repair itself. Within this context the question arises: Are there situations in which mechanisms can exhibit adaptive, self-corrective behavior or is the living organism something radically different from the rest of nature? If adaptive behavior is something manifested only by the living parts of nature, then they are in a sense outside the realm of the rest of nature. Yet we know that the basic structures of animate and inanimate matter are essentially the same.

Against this view, adaptive behavior is seen in a new perspective since the development of cybernetic theory.[19] With the development of cybernetic theory we can now understand how a mechanism can exhibit what we would regard as adaptive behavior. Such adaptive behavior exhibits certain patterns such as: (1) the system—organism or mechanism—is oriented toward some objective or target; (2) changes occur in the environment that tend to obstruct or impede the movement of the system toward its objective; (3) elements of the system are modified or regulated, whereby the impediment is evaded or overcome; and (4) normal movement toward the objective is resumed. Thus, a stone rolling down a hill is not an example of purposeful behavior. There is no purpose to its being at the bottom of the hill. But a rabbit coming out of its burrow and sensing the presence of a predator will exhibit purposeful behavior. It will sense the danger and adapt its actions accordingly. It will head underground once more. A dog trying to get into a fenced-in yard will also exhibit adaptive behavior. He may first walk around the perimeter of the fence looking for an opening. If none is found, he may try to climb over it or start digging underneath it. The actions of the rabbit and of the dog are examples of adaptive, target-oriented behavior.

Do mechanisms exhibit the same kind of behavior? Yes—if their material is organized in a certain way. For example, a thermostat system can be viewed as exhibiting target-oriented behavior. The thermostat is an automatic device for regulating temperature. It works by opening or closing the damper of a furnace in order to maintain a predetermined temperature. One way this is done is by utilizing the idea that different metals expand or contract at different rates during a temperature change. A loop composed of two different metals, like brass and steel, is fastened together with one end fixed and the other end attached to a pointer. If the surrounding temperature falls below the desired degree, the point bends to make contact with an electrical circuit, which is connected to an apparatus for opening the draft door of a furnace. When the temperature rises above the desired level, the pointer moves to make contact with another point until the circuit is closed and the draft door is closed.[20] The thermostat acts as a sensing device feeding information back to a part of this system that will respond accordingly.

If we confine our discussion to the province of the natural, then it is clear the developments in cybernetics have helped us to understand the natural structures and adaptive capacities of the living body. The term "natural" is not to be taken in some narrow sense of mechanistic materialism, but is intended to apply to all those events, things, and beings that may be investigated by the methods of the empirical sciences. In light of cybernetic theory, there are not two orders of being in nature. If inanimate material is organized in a certain way, then it will exhibit adaptive, self-corrective behavior as organic life does.

Most often adaptation or adaptive behavior is regarded as a modification or adjustment of the individual organism to bring it into accord with, or fitness for, the given environmental situation. However, adaptive behavior has a wider scope. It may involve not only a modification of the individual organism but also a more or less extensive transformation of its environment. Indeed, it would seem that the more advanced the life form or system is, the more likely it is to exhibit this second type of adaptive behavior, namely, the transformation of the environment to suit its needs. It is from such types of adaptation that the greatest benefits and the greatest evils of technological civilization have derived.

For some people, the idea of health may pertain only to the physiological mechanical system of the human body. For Dubos, it has a much wider significance. Concepts of health and disease refer not only to the individual body but also to the interaction between that individual and his environment—an environment that is social as well as physical. Just as the causes of disease may lie outside the skin of the human body, so their cure may require modification or regulation of those external environmental circumstances. Once this fact is recognized, it becomes evident that the adequate treatment of disease and the effective preservation of health entail the intervention of agencies that can control and regulate the physical and social environment. In other words, health in any comprehensive and enduring sense must become the responsibility of the community or the state. Private personal medicine and voluntary associations may accomplish much toward health, but they do not have the authority that alone can ensure an environment conducive to health. Health thereby becomes a communal or political undertaking. Medical science must, of course, help to supply the direction of policy but the effective application of this policy must ultimately rest on the authority of the community or government.

This social or political philosophy of medicine is not a challenge to medical science but to the traditional narrow range of its application. In the past, public health and social medicine have been peripheral auxiliaries of medical practice. If Dubos's philosophy gains acceptance, public health and social medicine will occupy more significant shares of medical practice. The focus of much of medicine is on its curative aspects, emphasizing the diagnosis and treatment of diseases. Such emphasis tends to exclude other aspects of medicine like public health and social medicine. Yet the late John Ryle, who was professor of clinical medicine at Cambridge and the first professor of social medicine at Oxford, noted years ago that "we no longer believe that medical truths are only or chiefly to be discovered under the microscope, by means of test tube and the animal experiment, or by chemical examination and increasingly elaborate pathological studies at the bedside."[21] By far the larger concern of medicine continues to be the individual specific treatment of complaints and disease. There is still only an avant-garde interest in a medical philosophy that sees man primarily in the context of his social and physical environment and conceives of health as depending on the interaction between the individual and that environment. Medical science needs to emphasize the importance of the study of the total environment where man is viewed as a part of it and not separate from it. This calls for the study of all factors that influence health, such as heredity, climate, occupation, and food. Without such an outlook, Dubos cautions, our efforts to remove social, economic, and physical evils may do more harm than good. The present emphasis on people as only physico-chemical systems ignores fundamental aspects of their nature. It obstructs the view of people as rational beings who are members of a family and a community with their well-being inextricably woven into the conditions of their home, their workplace, and their community.

Since there is no consensus on what constitutes health,[22] the total responsibility for the direction of policy related to health cannot be relegated solely to the nursing or medical professions. The collaboration of people from many different professional areas is needed.

Conclusion

Health, according to Dubos, is the state of effective and fruitful interaction of individuals with their constantly changing natural and social environments. The predominant feature of this interaction is adaptation. Within this context, disease is viewed as a failure in adaptation. However, freedom from signs and symptoms of disease does not mean that a state of health has been reached. Other types of deprivation, such as unsafe workplaces, lack of privacy, and excessive exposure to noise, may cause a breakdown in the adaptive responses of the individual. This also constitutes an unhealthy state.

Dubos delineated two kinds of adaptation: biological and social. Successful biological adaptation means that proper organic physicochemical mechanisms have been developed to cope with various environmental challenges. Far more important is the ability for social adaptation, as in successful interpersonal relationships. Dewey clarifies the concept of adaptation by distinguishing between passive adaptation and active adaptation. Adaptation is passive when the organism modifies itself to meet the requirements of the environment; adaptation is active when the organism modifies the environment to meet its needs. This view offers direction for social action. Adverse environmental conditions in communities are amenable to solution by altering such conditions. This is in contrast to the more conservative Social Darwinism, which views the individual as responsible for adapting to social conditions.

One of the important underlying ideas in the adaptive model is change. Dubos writes of the dynamic relationships between individuals and their environments. Thus, there are always demands for new kinds of adaptive behavior. The achievement of a stable condition of optimum health is viewed as impossible. What can be achieved is the development of adaptive responses in order to meet the continuous threats to health.

Implicit in this outlook is an ideal of human life by which its highest quality is attained through improved effectiveness and fruitfulness of this dynamic interaction between man and the environment. Such interaction marks the growth of the individual. The idea of growth formulated by Dewey is a clarifying concept for Dubos's work. According to Dewey, growth has biological, intellectual, and social components and refers to a steady expansion of one's abilities. Growth is life. One grows so that further growth is possible.

Chapter 8

EUDAIMONISTIC MODEL

This model comprises several views of human nature that extend the idea of health to general well-being and self-realization. This viewpoint is found in aspects of ancient Greek medicine and in the moral philosophies of Plato and Aristotle. The most significant modern representative of this conception of health is Abraham H. Maslow.[1] The idea of health developed in the writings of Maslow expresses a certain ideal of human nature and personality. It is the ideal of a person who can measure up to his wisest and best aspiration. The best aspiration is one that is directed to fulfillment and complete development. What is developed is the intrinsic potential. Health is the condition of actualization or realization of this potential.

Illness within this context is a condition that impedes or prevents this self-actualization. Treatment goes beyond the elimination of disease. The cure of a physiologic condition does not complete the task. One then has to aim at uncovering the "bent" of the individual's nature and assist him toward self-fulfillment.

Maslow has drawn a picture of an ideal of health that is both remarkable and strange. The path to health is a growing process and, once attained, results in good, joyful, creative human beings.

Healthy people, Maslow says, do not have to worry about their physiological functioning. All the conditions necessary for physical survival have been met. The healthy person not only has enough food, drink, and sleep to meet metabolic requirements and has shelter from the elements, he is also functioning at some optimal physiological level. But optimal physiologic functioning is only the first step on the road to health.

A person must also experience a sense of safety. He must feel protected and secure. The surrounding environment must be viewed as stable, manageable, predictable. The need to experience an orderly, carefree life is preferred over a chaotic, insecure lifestyle.

The healthy person will also want to experience love and affection, that feeling of being understood and appreciated for what one is. The healthy person trusts loved ones and can reveal weaknesses and faults without fear of losing another's love. He will also have the experience of being a member of a family or group. The healthy person will have a certain image of self and personality that engenders self-respect and self-confidence, which can, in turn, result in the respect, appreciation, and esteem of others toward him.

At this point, there will emerge something that the individual did not see as possible before—a certain refinement of sensibilities, enlarged vistas of experience, subtle refinements of all kinds (in music, art, literature, science, interpersonal relationships) that mark the epitome of the healthy, self-actualizing person.

Self-actualizing people, according to Maslow, share other common characteristics. Believing in an objective reality, Maslow thinks that healthy people have the potential of actually perceiving it. They can see life with all of its events and manifestations as it actually is and not filtered through their own subjective desires, beliefs, or fears.

Because of their ability to perceive reality correctly, self-actualizing people are able to see their own natures and the natures of others as they really are, remaining calm and imperturbable despite the deficiencies. There is self-acceptance in healthy people.

These people, along with being efficient in their perceptions of reality, are not afraid to deal with the uncertainties and ambiguities of life, and in fact will seek out those aspects of life that are hidden and mysterious, viewing them as challenging and exciting. They trust themselves and their perceptions of the world. They are spontaneous and creative and have the ability to live life to the fullest.

Many people would find this a strange idea. Tell a carpenter in his trade union about this conception of health and he would laugh. Tell him that he is not healthy and he would think you were crazy. "What do you mean," he might say. "I haven't seen a doctor for twenty years. And I've never been in a hospital." He arises at 7:00 A.M., has a healthy meal, and is at work by 8:00 A.M. He laughs and jokes with his co-workers, puts in a full eight-hour day with one-half hour off for lunch. He comes home—eats, has a beer, watches a few hours of television, and goes to bed. If Maslow saw this man he would say that he is not nearly as healthy as he could be. He has not begun to develop all that is necessary to be truly healthy.

A businessman goes to a physician for a check-up. His history, physical exam, blood work, x-rays, and all other studies are normal. The physician tells the man, "You are in wonderful shape. You're healthier than I am. Congratulations."

Maslow happens to overhear the conversation with a skeptical frown. "Healthy? What do you mean healthy? This man is far from the fullness of health of which he may be capable. He has barely begun to meet his lower needs. The business association has a very low opinion of him. His partners have abandoned him. He's viewed as a shyster and a crook. He comes home and there's no conversation with his wife because she hates him and he hates himself."

The doctor answers: "What are you talking about? Lower needs! His kidneys and abdomen are in fine shape. There's nothing wrong with them. No friends, no self-respect? My job isn't to teach him how to live. Let him go to his priest or rabbi. He's healthy as far as I'm concerned."

What is being argued is a question of morals—how one should lead a life. But the subtler question is: Can professional people be interested in health without having a set of values that describes human worth?

Mechanism and Holism

Maslow's viewpoint is an important idea attempting to redirect thinking away from a mechanistic view of man and toward a holistic view. It may be helpful at this point to distinguish between the idea of mechanism and the idea of holism.

The aim of all biological theory is to develop an adequate base for an understanding of the nature of life. Both the mechanistic and holistic theories in biology have this as their goal. In the mechanistic view of life, it is felt that all phenomena will turn out to be essentially material phenomena exhibiting causal relationships that follow the laws of mechanics. It is assumed that there are a limited number of laws governing the operation of these mechanical systems and once these laws are discovered, it becomes theoretically possible to understand every event that occurs within that mechanical system. Within this context, man is viewed as being a mechanistic organism where all of his activities, functions, structure, organization, and thoughts can be explained by the laws of mechanics.

J.H. Woodger outlines four meanings of the term "mechanism" that have been used to explain biological organisms, including man.[2] The first meaning uses the term as mechanical explanation in a very narrow sense, following the methods of classical mechanics. Living things exhibit the same laws that inorganic nature does. Physiologists holding this view say that all problems of life will be solved by a form of microscopic mechanical explanation of the physical organism.

The second use of the term treats the organism as being understood only if viewed in light of its physics and chemistry. Physical and chemical changes are viewed as the most basic of all changes in nature. This is based on the assumption that "the basis of life is an analyzable chemical compound or group of compounds" occurring at the cellular level.[3] Therefore, by concentrating on the physical and chemical studies of the processes that seem to constitute life, all that is important for the understanding of the nature of life can be gleaned from these kinds of experiments. What may seem to be initially unclear when using these experimental methods will, at some time in the future, prove to be understandable by the result of these same methods.

The third meaning of the term denotes the organism as machine-like. One group of thinkers adopts a dogmatic approach and views the organism as a machine and nothing beyond a machine. The other group of thinkers treats the organism as if it were a machine, saying that whatever the nature of the organism, we can understand it only if we think of it as a machine. This latter view does not make any statements about the ultimate nature of the organism. This view strives to overcome the defects of the physico-chemical view of a mechanism, which does not address itself to the question of wholeness. This view does attempt to look at the whole organism. The human being is seen as being composed of parts but also as an individual entity—a whole equal to the sum of its parts.

The fourth use of the term involves causal explanations. This means that the life processes are viewed as proceeding in an orderly way, "producing similar effects under similiar conditions."[4]

In order to discover the underlying mechanical laws that govern the organism's vital processes, the organism must be viewed in terms of its components. Experiments are set up so that the part being studied can be isolated from the whole and is exposed to only one stimulus at a time. For example, in the study of muscle contractility in the frog, the muscle that is tested is completely removed from the frog's leg and hooked to the kymograph. This procedure is an example of what has been called the method of mechanistic analysis, which was initiated by the seventeenth-century French philosopher René Descartes. The central feature of this method is the postulate that (a) any whole can be analyzed into parts that can be isolated such that (b) the characteristics of these parts can be investigated in isolation from the whole, and (c) from the characteristics of the parts, the properties of the whole can be inferred.[5]

This mechanistic view has added to our understanding of living organisms. For example, we know quite a lot about reflexes, the difference between sensory and motor activity of the nervous system, the sympathetic nervous system, and the effects of the ductless glands on the body.[6]

Other examples of mechanistic views of phenomena above the subsystem level of the organism follow. For example, the human being is viewed as being constituted of "dormant" reflexes waiting to be activated by specific physical stimuli. These reflexes, activated over the course of the organism's life by stimuli from both the organism and the environment, form a series of mechanisms we call habits. The reflexes, their reaction to stimuli, and the formation of habits within the organism are seen as "physico-chemical modifications of the nervous system."[7] "That which we call 'mind' and its activities (thinking, understanding) are viewed as complex movements within the brain, nervous system or other bodily organs."[8] Hunger, thirst, and sexual desires are experienced because, machine-like, we are compelled to do so.[9] That which is called an idea may eventually be found to cause chemical changes in the body, thereby providing a mechanistic explanation for why certain people are willing to die for a cause.[10]

The method of mechanistic analysis has been very fruitful for science. As a matter of fact, this method is the foundation upon which science, as we know it, has been built.

Some results of the application of the method of mechanistic analysis to biology are:

1. The development and growth of the fields of anatomy, physiology, biochemistry, embryology, bacteriology, psychology.
2. The isolation and identification of proteins, fats, and carbo-

hydrates; the study of the process of digestion; colloid-ion-enzyme chemistry; carbon and nitrogen cycles.

Because of the fruitfulness of the Cartesian world view with its method of mechanistic analysis in understanding natural phenomena, biologists felt that it was only a matter of time before full understanding of the nature of life would be attained. But research activities have generated many more questions than they have answered.

Some investigators allege that there appear to be several kinds of biological phenomena that cannot be explained by the method of mechanistic analysis. Two examples of these biological phenomena include: (1) an explanation of the function of the brain regarding feelings, emotions, and abstract thought, and (2) an adequate explanation regarding the origins of life. How did the first organisms arise? There is very little useful scientific information on this topic. The scarcity of fruitful theories to explain such phenomena has led some researchers to develop alternative doctrines regarding the nature of life. One such doctrine that is opposed to the mechanistic conception of life is the holistic conception, widely accepted in contemporary biology.

William McDougall defines "holistic." It is "the name for a group of similar theories which seeks to explain the nature of life by insisting upon the wholeness, unity, and individuality of each organism as a characteristic which must be taken into account by every attempt to explain the vital processes,"[11] such as consciousness, adaptation, growth, and reproduction.

The characteristics of wholeness, unity, and individuality of the organism become assumptions upon which this biology is based. Other formulations of the idea have been advanced:

1. The organism is a whole and a whole is more than the sum of its parts.
2. The whole exhibits emergent (i.e., new) properties and modes of action and these are therefore unpredictable.
3. The whole has a unity, organization, and individuality that is not discoverable by means of the analysis of its parts. In fact, the analysis of the parts of the organism results in decreased perceptions of the qualities of the whole.
4. The whole controls, dominates, and directs the formation of its parts, although the parts also influence the whole.[12]

McDougall distinguishes two different modes of thought among those accepting the concept of holism. One is the organismic biological doctrine (also called organismic theory, organicism, organismal conception of life) associated with, among others, Ludwig von Bertalanffy and Kurt Goldstein. The other is the doctrine of teleological holism held by such men as J.B.S. Haldane, A.N. Whitehead, and Jan C. Smuts.

Both of the aforementioned groups accept the notion of holism. Both groups reject the idea of mechanism, although most of the organismic biologists regard their view as consistent with eventual explanations in terms of physico-chemical concepts. On the other hand, teleological holism is opposed to any kind of mechanistic explanation. Only the ideas of Bertalanffy and Goldstein will be presented.

Bertalanffy states his disagreement with the mechanistic conception of life. He says that "mechanism provides us with no grasp of the specific characteristics of organisms, of the organization of organic processes among one another, of organic 'wholeness,' of the problem of the origin of organic 'teleology,' or of the historical character of organisms."[13]

The mechanistic outlook, says Bertalanffy, fails to account for fundamental adaptive and self-serving roles of the organism.

> Whether we consider nutrition, voluntary and instinctive behavior, development, the harmonious functioning in cases of disturbances of the normal, we find that all vital processes are so organized that they are directed to the maintenance [each organ performing functions necessary to the upkeep of the organism], production, or restoration of the wholeness of the organism. On that account the physicochemical description of the vital processes [is not exhaustive].[14]

For Bertalanffy, the task of biology is to discover the laws of biological systems to which the ingredient parts and processes are subordinate.[15]

Kurt Goldstein, the distinguished neurologist and researcher, supports his holistic views by observations of various neurological phenomena involving people with brain and other nervous system injuries. According to Goldstein, his investigations raise fundamental questions concerning the adequacy of mechanistic explanations of the living being. Goldstein views physico-chemical processes as playing no greater part than other phenomena of the organism."[16] He does not accept the thesis that examination of the physico-chemical processes of the organism will result in the formulation of the nature of the whole organism.

How can the following events be explained by a mechanistic conception of life, he asks. He described one of his brain-injured patients who could read only if each letter presented to him was on a line. If the letter was on an unlined page, the patient could not read it. If the patient drew a line under the letter, he could read immediately.[17]

Other patients, who were aphasic and had simultaneous injury of speech and reading centers of the brain, when asked to read aloud would not necessarily understand what they had to read. But the same patients could read with full understanding if they did so silently. Patients failed in their tasks, which they could otherwise do, if the requested performance involved the same injured areas of the brain.[18]

He also learned that any aspect of the body that can emulate writing movements can be used to write without any previous training. This shift occurs without undue effort when the ability to write in the usual way is no longer possible, as when due to some injury or disease.

Goldstein also cites a number of neurological studies that show that changes in any part of an organism produce measurable changes in any part of that organism the experimenter chose to test. For example, one group of muscles can be stimulated and electrical changes in corresponding muscle groups can be demonstrated, as when an action current in the muscles of the foot flexors was found when the fingers were flexed.[19]

Because of such experimental results, he finally rejects mechanistic explanations and accepts holism. He says that the explanations of all experiments that were carried out to adduce evidence that the preferences of the organism are based on the interplay of individually separate phenomena are unsuitable. "To attempt to understand life from the point of view of the natural science method alone is fruitless."[20]

While Bertalanffy speaks of the system as being the organism's most important quality, Goldstein writes that the constancy of the organism is the basis upon which to build the idea of wholeness. He feels that the organism, despite all variations in behavior and despite all the changes that occur during a lifetime, retains a stability by which it is possible to maintain organismic identity as a structural form. This constancy, this stability, is the essence of the organism.

McDougall points out that there are many biological findings that cannot be explained by the holistic doctrines. These findings show that parts of the organism do in fact function apart from the whole. So the whole cannot in all cases influence the parts. McDougall outlines some of these findings, citing two examples.

> The development of sarcomas and cancers seems to illustrate [such] successful rebellion of parts. The cultivation of a piece of tissue in vitro is difficult to reconcile with the holistic principle. W.H. Gaskell showed that an isolated strip of heart muscle may continue to "beat" for many hours. . . . A. Carrell and others have shown that bits of tissue may grow indefinitely in suitable media and conditions. Even an eye-rudiment may develop almost normally in vitro.[21]

It would seem that in light of this discussion the methods of both doctrines are useful in studying the nature of life. Both are true within their own context. Neither one will result in complete understanding of nature and human nature.

The method selected for analysis will be determined by the nature of the questions raised. For example, if one raises questions about man's behavior, then the whole person can be studied in relation to a series of environmental stimuli. But studying the behavioral manifestations of the person will tell us nothing about the details of cellular, tissue, or organic structure and function. However, dissecting the human body and studying its parts will tell us a great deal about these matters, but nothing about that body's behavior. Thus, our knowledge of the human organism will be incomplete if we study only the parts or only the characteristics of the whole.

Crick shows how the study of both the whole and its parts apply to all the fields in biology. The biological system, he says, can be viewed as a hierarchy of levels of organization where the wholes of one level are the parts of the next. Therefore, cells are the wholes of cellular biology but the parts of tissue biology, which are the parts of organ biology, and so on.[22]

Critique of Maslow's Work

M. Brewster Smith is one of a number of psychologists who has written critically about Maslow's concept of self-actualization.[23] One target of Smith's criticism is the way in which Maslow arrived at his conception of the self-actualizing person. For Maslow, the self-actualizing person is the healthy person. The question Smith asks is:

How does Maslow arrive at his concept of health? How does Maslow select the people whom he considers healthy?

In order to arrive at a general concept of health, Maslow observed people around him and he also studied the backgrounds and personalities of notable public and historical figures, looking for those people whom he felt were in the process of making full use of their talents, abilities, potentialities. It is this condition of wholeness and fulfillment that Maslow calls health. He finally selected nine contemporaries and nine historical figures who, he thought, were healthy people in this sense. By direct observation of his contemporaries and by biographical studies of historical figures, he sought to arrive at those general traits of personality that would characterize this group in particular and other "healthy" people in general. These studies served as part of the basis for his conception of the self-actualizing person.

Smith views Maslow's method of selecting self-actualizing people as a "crucial flaw" in his work. He says that Maslow "eliminated people with gross pathology—the Dostoevskis and Van Goghs—and selected people for whom . . . he had the highest admiration as human specimens. His empirical definition of psychological health or self-actualization thus rests, at root, on his own implicit values that underlie this global judgment."[24]

Smith makes two points about Maslow's work. First, he says that Maslow has made a choice; he has shown a preference for people who exhibit certain characteristics that he thinks exemplify health. Second, Smith points out that the qualities Maslow says characterize the healthy person may not be the qualities anybody else would choose in developing a general conception of health—the qualities Maslow chose are peculiar to Maslow. While this may be true, it does not negate Maslow's approach.

If a gardener wanted to identify the best quality rose, he would look for the best example of that species, one that he felt had all of the qualities necessary for the title Best Rose. He would want to study that particular rose; subjectively look at it, smell it before he would decide that it is superior to all the other roses that he has seen and smelled. He would then carefully study that rose again, along with the bush that produced it, the soil that it grew in, and the climate that enveloped it until he identified those qualities of the bush, soil, and climate that produced that best-of-all-possible roses. Then he would want to replicate those same conditions so that more bushes would produce good roses.

The same procedure can be followed in identifying healthy

people. Determine the kinds of qualities associated with healthy people; look at people who can be considered healthy; see what qualities they have and how they got that way. The qualities identified through this kind of inquiry can be considered standards of health. This is what Maslow chose to do, proceeding in much the same way as that gardener. Maslow used the term *iteration* to describe his method. It is a helical process, which is circular and involves a progression, like a spiral. Thus, his investigations were not lineal.

Maslow also used medicine as a model for his work but went beyond it. In medicine, in order to determine the optimal functioning of organ-systems in people, the organs people should normally have are identified and their functioning is determined. People who have all of their bodily organs intact and functioning the way they should are considered physiologically healthy. But Maslow says that physiologic health is not enough. Man is more than a physiologic organism; he is a social being. He needs more than optimal physiologic functioning before he can be considered healthy. He needs to feel safe, secure, free from anxiety. He needs to have the love of those close to him and feel part of a group. And he needs to love in return. He also needs the respect of others and has to have a sense of his own value. When these basic needs are met, he will start growing in all kinds of ways that he may not have thought possible. It is the people who exhibit these kinds of characteristics that Maslow calls healthy.

He correctly eliminated people from his sample who exhibited gross pathology. He wanted examples of healthy people. Van Gogh and, to a lesser degree, Dostoevsky, according to his criteria, were not healthy people. Maslow never said that sick people could not paint superb pictures or write great novels, but he did say that if talented, creative people are morose, suicidal (as Van Gogh was), wretched, and they make other people suffer, then they are not healthy people nor are they leading healthy lives.

The identification of top-quality characteristics of the healthy rose or healthy person is dependent on the good judgment of the observer. When selecting the standard of health of roses or people, observer perceptions must be accurate. What the observer perceives as being characteristics of health in people or roses should find agreement among others also. Who would object to the list of qualities that Maslow has generated in order to identify the self-actualizing person—qualities such as wholeness, self-sufficiency, justice, beauty, honesty, grace, joy? These would certainly represent the highest and best qualities of which human beings are capable.

Smith's criticisms of Maslow's methods of selecting his sample of self-actualizing people lead to a basic question: How does anyone decide who is healthy? Maslow, who was interested in identifying people who were preeminently healthy, selected people for study who had the qualities and characteristics that he thought characterized the healthy person. Far from being invalid, this may be the way all concepts of health are generated. Maslow, however, is explicit in his approach. Generally, the development of concepts of health are more implicit.

It is possible that any analysis of the question, "what do people think health is," will show that these concepts of health have a moral foundation—moral in the sense that health is one among other values by which we conceive the ideal person. It is on this moral foundation that cultural tradition is based.

Anthropolgical and sociological studies have disclosed numerous instances of cultural diversity when dealing with the recognition of a condition as health, or illness. Depending on the level of social and economic development within a culture, the standard of health can be very low. In many societies, signs and symptoms of disease are commonplace and are accepted as the norm rather than viewed as abnormal. Therefore, most people who are functioning are not necessarily physiologically well.

Conditions of the body that in Western European culture would at once be identified as illness are treated as normal healthy states among some people of the world. Such disparities have been reported even among different economic and educational strata of technologically advanced societies. For example, Koos reports in a study of an upper New York state town that when presented with a list of seventeen medically important symptoms, members of the upper social stratum would tend to think of themselves as ill when experiencing these symptoms, while they would be generally disregarded by members of the lower social stratum.[25]

Since the healthy condition is often identified as the norm, illnesses that are present at a high prevalence in a population tend to be regarded as normal, tolerable, and a kind of healthy condition. For example, Strole et al., in their study of residents of mid-Manhattan, showed that when using their criteria of impairment and readiness for professional help, the people who never received psychiatric care seemed unlikely to seek professional help of their own accord while health professionals felt that a large potential demand for intervention existed.[26]

The events and activities of our daily lives become so commonplace that most of us rarely maintain our curiosity about them. It is only after our usual patterns of activity are interfered with that questions regarding our condition are raised. Interviews with ninety-five people, aged sixty-five and over who lived in a low socioeconomic area of Boston, showed that they thought of health only if they perceived it as poor health, i.e., illness. They had minimal conceptions of what health was. Health was viewed as the ability to eat, sleep, keep going[27]—as the ability to function in work and play without being hampered by their physical condition. This conception of health is seen as the absence of malfunctioning. The norm is the ability to carry out accustomed activities. People generally establish norms by calling certain conditions "malfunctioning" if what is generally expected is not done. When they cannot do what is generally expected, then people are considered to be unhealthy.

One conception of health that seems to profoundly influence American society is the Calvinist conception of the healthy man as one who does his duty and does his work; he does that which is required of him. Early American Puritanism was an expression of this Calvinist doctrine of personal salvation. The Puritans held the notion that life was to be conducted in a specific ethical way in order to attain salvation. While salvation can never be attained by performing good works, the performance of good works can make man's soul more amenable to receiving God's grace. In order to be deserving of God's grace, Puritans considered certain qualities to be moral virtues and these were incorporated into their patterns of life. These virtues centered around serious work and practical achievement and included discipline, frugality, industry, moderation, and simplicity.[28] The influence of this Puritan ethic, based upon Calvinist moral doctrines, was felt far beyond the Massachusetts Bay area. The high level of morality that resulted from adherence to this moral doctrine helped shape the ethics of our culture. One of the results of this moral doctrine was the development within our society of the concept of work as an indispensable part of man's life. While the healthy man is viewed as one who is doing his work, a man would be considered ill if he is not able to fulfill the normal expectations of work and duty.

Culture on a higher level of civilization cultivates values that go far beyond simple economic, social, and religious factors or role expectations. These higher values deal with the development of an ideal of human worth—the ideal of a person who can measure up to his wisest and his best aspiration. This is what Maslow had in mind and what the early Greeks in the age of Plato envisioned. Health within this context is thought of as embracing qualities of more subtle forms: development of art, literature, science; the capacity to enjoy life and contribute effectively to the quality of life of others; continual and creative growth of all our sensibilities.

As these few illustrations indicate, ideas of health are generally expressions of values that form part of a culture pattern of people. These values are not usually made explicit but they function as implicit norms within the society. Maslow's conception of health, unlike these other conceptions, is made explicit but is no more "invalid" or slanted than the health ideals of other cultural traditions, nor can it be said that these ideas are peculiar to Maslow. In many respects they are expressions of the eudaimonic traditions of Plato and Aristotle.

Smith's criticism is also concerned with Maslow's conception of human potentialities. Maslow is using the term potentiality to refer to human traits such as creativity, ethical conduct, grace, and joy. These are traits inherent in the human being that are capable of further development and growth, and it is in this sense that Maslow is using the term.

Concerning this idea of human potentialities, Smith says that "the young person has an extremely broad range of multiple potentialities. The course of life . . . excludes some of them, sets limits on others, and elaborates upon still others. Vice and evil are as much in the range of human potentiality . . . as virtue."[29]

There seems to be an equivocation here with the word potentiality. In Smith's criticism potentiality is used in the sense of possibility. This is a fundamental error. The idea of the potentiality of a living organism derives from the conception of some ideal or perfected form of that organism. On the other hand, the idea of possibility bears no such relation to the perfection of the species. When an acorn grows into an oak it is actualizing its potentiality. But it would be a travesty to say that the acorn is fulfilling its potentiality when it is eaten by an animal. Likewise, it is absurd to speak of vice and evil as the potentiality of a human being. Vice and evil are so called precisely because they frustrate or destroy human potentiality. There are wide ranges of possibilities for all of us. A young woman, showing great skill as a union organizer, becomes an alcoholic and barbiturate addict, thereby destroying a range of her potentialities. This is why we want to avoid these kinds of destructive habits. We all have possibilities for vice and evil within us, but we want to cultivate our potentialities in order to avoid the negative possibilities.

People can use their human traits for good or evil. The acute observational abilities, analytic capacities, and intelligence that can lead a physiology researcher to break the genetic code can also be

applied to war strategies or bank robberies. The use of human intelligence in these ways does not negate Maslow's use of the word
potentiality for the development and growth of those traits that
characterize the active, mature person.

The term potentiality implies that there is personal growth. The
capacity for personal growth is continuous. There is no end to it. We
grow so that we can grow some more.[30] Maslow's idea of potentiality
is based on the biological model of growth, for example, the conditions attending the growth of an acorn into an oak tree. An acorn falls
to the ground and under proper conditions it will grow into a full,
living oak tree. When this happens, the acorn is fulfilling its nature.
But the development and growth of this acorn into an oak tree is not
all of its possibilities. It can be eaten by an animal; it can be pierced,
strung on a string, and worn as a necklace; it can be hollowed out and
used as a pipe in play. These are some of the possibilities of the
acorn, but the interesting thing is that none of the possibilities fulfills its nature. In these possibilities, the entire structure and ingredients of the acorn are not completely utilized. In eating the acorn,
only certain parts of the material would be absorbed into the animal's
system. The organization of the acorn as a seed does not enter into
the nourishment of the animal. Consequently, only some of its chemical ingredients are utilized. Drilling a hole through it does not alter
its frame, but its function is interfered with. Hollowing it out de-
stroys its internal pattern. These uses are not fulfilling its nature.
Only the partial character of the acorn is utilized in these examples.
The only use that will ensure full development of its inherent potential is to have it take root in the earth and grow into an oak tree.
When it functions as a seed, all of its nature participates. It is in this
sense that Maslow is using the term potentiality—to denote the fullest development and growth of all of which we are capable.

The adult human being can create systems of science and works of
art. These are coordinated with other human traits: prehensile
hands, speech, skillful use of tools. Maslow refers to incipient forms
of these traits in the infant, child, and young person. We can expose
the infant to conditions in which these traits are frustrated. We can
also expose him to congenial conditions in which these traits will
blossom, like the oak tree did when the acorn took root. Human
beings, under the proper conditions, will develop their intelligence,
analytic skills, courage, and aesthetic senses. In Maslow's sense, this
development is the actualization of their potentialities. Growth as
used here is not to be viewed as the idea of quantitative extension as
when pouring water into a column of glass, resulting in first an inch

of water, then two inches of water, and three inches of water. Growth here is used in the sense of development of functions, power, and freedom.

Smith also says that our potentialities as viewed by Maslow are predetermined, as in the Aristotelian sense. Man has these potentialities within him in rudimentary forms. The environment has no part in determining what these rudimentary potentialities are, although the environment will help to influence the ranges of potentialities that will become actualized. While in agreement with Smith's interpretation of Maslow's idea, Maslow's views do not negate evolutionary modification. While a "tiger becomes tigerish or a horse more equine," organisms can and do change in response to environmental conditions. For example, a certain species of moth exists in industrial, polluted areas of England and in relatively unpolluted parts of the country. In the heavily industrial area, the moth that predominates has dark coloring and therefore blends in with the soot that covers the trees. In unpolluted areas, its lighter colored forms predominate. These moths still are "mothish," but certain phenotypes, developed via genetic processes, survive longer because of these evolutionary color changes. The survivors are better camouflaged from their predators.

People can be seen as changing also, despite their inherent potentialities. At this stage of our development where we are seen as social beings, the self-actualization traits that Maslow has outlined are the highest qualities of which we are capable. But we can continue to evolve other qualities, ones that we might want to include as self-actualizing characteristics—such as telepathic ability, which we have not yet shown as existing in human nature. It could, one day, be considered a desirable part of human nature and outstanding enough to be considered among self-actualizing characteristics.

Conclusion

Within the context of the eudaimonistic model, health is the condition of complete development of the individual's potential. Illness is the condition that interrupts or obstructs this development.

The eudaimonistic model furnishes a more extensive conception of health because it can be viewed as focusing on the entire nature of the individual: physical, social, aesthetic, and moral, instead of just certain aspects of human behavior and physiology. Maslow explicitly incorporates into his ideal of health the best qualities of which man is capable. As such, this conception of health can be viewed as marking the epitome of the civilized person. To be healthy in the eudaimonistic sense is a goal to aim for, a value worth striving for. Health within the context of the other models can be viewed as constituting a basis from which to build toward the cultured, uplifting traits of the eudaimonistic model of health.

Maslow has argued for a very high level of health. He has written about an ideal of human worth and, in this sense, his work is parallel to the moral philosophies of Plato, Aristotle, and Hippocractic medicine.

Chapter 9

STRUCTURE AND INTERRELATIONSHIPS OF THE FOUR MODELS

The four models of health presented here can be viewed as alternative ideas of health, although they are not mutually exclusive ideas. The adoption of one model does not preclude the adoption of the other models of health, although the degree of emphasis put on each model may differ. But they can also be viewed as forming a scale—a progressive expansion of the idea of health. The models of health can be seen as viewing individuals within broader and broader contexts.

The narrowest view, the clinical model, views individuals within the boundary of their skin. They are seen as physiologic systems with interrelated functions. Health within this context is viewed as the absence of signs and symptoms of derangement within the physiologic or body-mind system. Illness constitutes signs and symptoms of disease, derangement, or malfunctioning of the body or mind. This constitutes a negative conception of health because it emphasizes the idea of illness, not health. This model suggests the characteristics of diseases. If a person does not have a disease, then he or she is considered healthy. The physician's job is to certify the human organism as physiologically sound. There is little concern on the part of the physician with what happens to the patient outside the office. Nevertheless, the clinical model is a fundamentally important concept because it is a minimal idea of health. Within the context of the clinical model, a person who has the signs and symptoms

of disease can never be considered healthy regardless of how productive or creative he is. If a person is considered healthy even
though signs and symptoms of disease are present, then another
standard of health is being used.

The other models of health add additional requirements to this
idea of health because they do not focus on clinical illness, but rather
concentrate on the more positive qualities of life. Thus, to be healthy
one has to at least meet the standards of the clinical model. But these
standards are not enough if some positive aspects to health are to be
introduced.

Next on the scale is the idea of health as role-performance. This is
an advance beyond the clinical model because it adds a social-
psychological standard to the idea of health. Persons need to be not
only physiologically sound in the clinical sense but also socially fit.
The role-performance model, while not rejecting the clinical conception of health, conceives the idea of health in a wider perspective,
involving the complex of social relationships and functions into
which people enter because of their roles. From this viewpoint,
people who find their social niche and fulfill their social roles
adequately are healthy. Failure in role-performance may mean illness, even if people are clinically healthy. They may fail because they
have not developed adequate social-psychological traits. On the
other hand, adequate role-performance may not be sufficient. A person may perform well in his role as an accountant but not in his role
as a father. Besides, social circumstances are not fixed. Changes in a
community precipitate changed roles and this demands a capacity for
change, for flexible adaptation—a requirement that goes beyond
mere role-performance.

The adaptive model is more expansive than the other two but
incorporates them. People within this context not only have to be
physiologically healthy and perform their roles adequately, but they
must also show adaptive behavior—the creative adjustment to
changing circumstances. It expresses growth, expansion, and creativity. The routine, inflexible life of the role-performance model is in-
sufficient for health in this sense. This model generalizes the idea of
people and their health by viewing them as adaptive systems in
relation to their social and natural environments.

The most comprehensive and expansive conception of health is
the eudaimonistic model, which extends the idea of people and their
health to embrace capacities and activities in science, art, religion,
and other enterprises of culture. Maslow described the ideal: the
self-actualizing, fulfilled and fulfilling, loving personality. Thus, the

eudaimonistic model is the most comprehensive because it embraces the three preceding models in the series.

From another viewpoint, these four ideas of health appear as four ideals of humanity. The clinical model views individuals as physiologic systems and the role-performance model views individuals as elements in the social fabric. The adaptive model sees the ideal people as flexible, effective participants in a challenging environment that they are capable of meeting by means of their adaptive resources. Finally, the eudaimonistic concept presents an ideal of the civilized, cultured person who has the capacity for continuous growth, the refinement of sensibilities, and creativity.

Implications of the Models of Health

Health is a directive aim in the practice of the nurse and other professions interested in it. Four significant directive ideas of health have been identified and analyzed. Thus, four different targets at which the nurse can aim have been provided. Nurses will direct their practices in light of whatever model is adopted. Each model, that is, each target, leads to different goals.

The differences among the four models of health do not entail opposition; all four have a certain fundamental validity in relation to human needs and aspirations. Nevertheless, there are certain significant differences in outlook and emphasis. The clinical and role-performance models on the one hand and the adaptive and eudaimonistic models on the other appear in very different perspectives. Both the clinical and role-performance models seem focused on the maintenance of stability; they may be said to aim at physiologic and social homeostasis. In contrast, the adaptive and eudaimonistic models are oriented toward change and growth.

The Clinical Model: Fundamental to Nursing Practice

Practice within the scope of the clinical model has been primarily concerned with the cure and prevention of diseases, with the knowledge to treat disease based on the study of the biological and physical sciences. People with various psychological and physiologic problems present themselves to a physician, whose job is to help them understand the nature of their problems and the methods available in treating or curing them. Medical practice thus emphasizes the elimination of the physical and mental conditions of disease and the alleviation of any accompanying pain. Interest in the cure and control of disease has become the predominant interest of the medical profession.

Most nursing school curricula (based on the authority of the physician) show an intensive concern with various diseases, their treatment, and the nursing care specific to these diseases. During their course of study, student nurses become preoccupied with the care and treatment of the sick, most of whom are in hospital settings. More specifically, they become focused on a specific subsystem that is acutely diseased and this concern in maintained after graduation. For example, a nurse caring for an arthritic admitted to the hospital for pneumonia generally does not instruct that person in the range-of-motion exercises that will maintain a preadmission level of functioning. Without such instruction, a person returning home from the hospital, after being immobile and bedridden, may no longer be able to perform some of the usual activities of daily living like combing one's hair and climbing stairs. Disuse of arthritic joints leads to decreased mobility of those joints.

Although there is a growing awareness that health care should embrace the whole person, the rewards still lie in other, more specialized directions. Those at the top of the nursing hierarchy in hospitals are still the specialists (enterostomal therapists, respiratory specialists), whose knowledge and professional interests are concentrated on small parts of the human body. It is, in other words, the clinical model that informs nursing education and research, as well as the general practice of nurses and physicians. Both are focused on the control and elimination of specific disease symptoms.

This is not said in opposition to the clinical model but only in recognition of its limitations. Whatever these limitations are, the clinical model remains the fundamental pattern of health care. It is this pattern of curative medicine that has shaped the traditions of the modern nursing profession. The high reputation of that profession still rests on the performance of the traditional nurse—that combination of skilled service and compassionate dedication that has been the image of the classical nurse. This nurse, unlike the physician, is the person who maintains direct physical contact with the patient in administering care and in performing essential observations. In this nurse one finds competent professional knowledge united with personal service. This nurse has, together with scientific training, the special talents of sensitivity, empathy, and the capacity to manifest affectionate concern, as well as the skill for imparting reassurance, confidence, and hope.

In 1980, approximately two-thirds of the total active nursing population of 1.3 million were employed in hospitals.[1] Most of the physicians, whose education and training are also based on the clinical model, are in hospital settings, and they have control over the delivery of the kind of services implicit in the clinical model. Consequently, the majority of nurses are employed in settings where physicians in large part determine their scope of practice.

Can the Nursing Role Be Expanded Within the Clinical Model?

Recent discussions of the science and practice of medicine have been increasingly critical of what is here called the clinical model.[2] It is said that with their present orientation, nurses and physicians, even if they deliver more of the same kinds of services, are not going to significantly improve the health of the population.

> There have been no significant improvements in the public's health in recent years except for a small decline in the incidence of heart disease, attributable in large measure to improved diet and more exercise. At the margin, medical care appears to have stopped making a difference. Medical care aids many individuals in restoring and maintaining their health, but significant improvements in the overall health levels of the population are not being achieved through its provision.[3]

The clinical model implies little concern for the future. The patients present themselves and are treated. There is little thought to what happens outside of the hospital or clinic, whereas the other three models cannot escape the relation of the person to the larger environment.

Despite such reports of the impact of medical care on health, discussions in nursing journals and conferences[4] have shown an increasing interest in the expansion of the role of nursing into areas traditionally designated by law as the physician's domain. These expanded role areas include the diagnosis and treatment of minor acute illnesses and management of chronic stable conditions by the nurse, who is nevertheless still under the "supervision" of the physician. This is a vital issue that affects the education of nurses as well as the practice of nursing because it clearly shows an increasing dependence on the physician and continuing acceptance of the narrow concept of health as delineated in the clinical model. But if this kind of practice is a viable alternative for nurses, then we must be able to decide such issues as whether there are areas of medical diagnosis and treatment in which a nurse can be qualified to make independent judgments; areas that extend beyond the limits of current practice now imposed upon nurses by law.

Certainly professional status implies the ability to make autonomous judgments and exercise discretion in practice. In order to progress toward professionalization by means of the expanded role, we must be able to clearly specify the areas of decision for which the nurse is qualified to practice independently, and those areas in which the nurse is limited to pursuing activities stipulated by the supervising doctor. If we can delineate these areas, then we can try to make them a legal part of independent nursing practice.

With regard to the foregoing issues, we need to determine to what extent a nurse with a traditional education and training can practice medical diagnosis and therapy. The nurse is clearly not qualified to make all medical diagnoses or institute all therapy without further education and training. In other words, we need clear formulations of how, with the present education, the nurse's role can be expanded.

If it seems that the professionalization of nurses requires a new educational program, then we must determine what curriculum can be provided for post-registered nurse training that will enable the nurse to function as an independent, autonomous nurse practitioner. Presently, post-registered nurse training seems to be without professional standardization or regulation. Programs vary widely in areas of content, practice requirements, duration, and rigor. Nurse practitioners who, on the basis of such informal post-registered nurse training, have expanded their activities into some areas of professional medicine (even if under the supervision of a physician), have been challenged in the courts.

It is clear that such proposals for professional nursing practice require the development of curriculum and training standards approved by the nursing and medical professions and signalized by some kind of thorough, formal post-registered nurse certification or professional degree. Until this technical education is put on such sound basis, decisions regarding independence and autonomy of nurses practicing certain aspects of traditional medicine will not be possible.

Such decisions will have to consider other options in the future development of the nursing profession. Instead of more intensive training within the clinical model, there are new areas of knowledge and practice indicated by the adaptive and eudaimonistic models.

The expansion in these directions is not an invasion of the physician's role but constitutes the assumption of distinctively new responsibilities for the nursing profession.

If we aim for the professionalization of the nurse by means of the expanded role in areas of medical practice, who is going to maintain physical contact with the patient? Presumably, the new nurse-practitioner, in assuming some of the functions of the physician, will surrender the traditional functions of nursing to some other health care worker—perhaps the practical nurse or the orderly. This raises a new question: Is the need for this new practitioner sufficient to justify the loss of the classical nursing role?

We should scrutinize the nature and magnitude of the need for the expanded-role nurse in medical practice. The question of need should of course be distinguished from other aspects of the proposal for a new role, such as the alleged enhanced dignity and the supposed economic advancement of the nurse. The need that is being addressed is the community's need. Who needs the expanded-role nurses and where are they needed? Clearly a need has been established in areas where communities have been unable to maintain the services of a physician—rural areas and inner-city ghettos. But in relation to the total number of nurses in the United States, the number of such positions where one would perform some primary care functions with only remote supervision from a physician is very small. If the education of expanded-role nurses is designed to meet these needs, it may not have to grow into an extraordinarily massive movement in order to accomplish a limited task.

The foregoing comments are not designed to oppose the proposed expansion of the role of the nurse into curative medicine. They are offered only as suggestions for further scrutiny—to invite attention to some problems that confront such an undertaking.

Health Care: The Distinctive Nursing Role Under the Adaptive and Eudaimonistic Models

Increasing attention is being focused on the distinction between the medical care of the clinical model and what is called health care. It is becoming increasingly recognized that medical care is not synonymous with health care. To put it less paradoxically, there are different kinds of health care and they differ depending on the model of health upon which they are predicated. What has been traditionally designated as medical care is oriented toward what is here called the clinical concept of health. The difference between this and the other models of health is, in one respect, a matter of range of concern and activity, with the clinical model being the narrowest in that it is intensively and almost exclusively focused on the physical and psychological functioning of the organism. To say this is not to denigrate this model of health or the medical and nursing care directed by it. It is simply to state its characteristic feature and to distinguish it from other kinds of health care centered on the other models of health. If the clinical model is narrow, it is nevertheless essential. No other model can be adequate without the concerns of the clinical model.

The primary concern of the medical doctor—the identification, cure, and, to some extent, the prevention of disease—must be an indispensable part of any health care. Diagnosis and treatment of disease are what people seek and what physicians are especially trained for. People's lives, however, are part of a complex nexus of relations: economic, social, political, and emotional; they have "problems" touching this intricate social fabric. These are not within the purview of the clinical model. In this model illness is conceived in terms of specific complaints pertaining to pains and malfunctions of the body and, accordingly, the medical care in the clinical model is aimed at the specific signs and symptoms linked to these complaints. These problems may have a special urgency and attention to them may be fundamental, but those other problems affecting the quality of life may demand almost equal attention in the other models of health.

While the cure and control of disease have become the primary interests of the medical doctor, it is notable that most of the improvements in standards of health have developed outside curative medicine. They have resulted from public health measures and socioeconomic changes. Mortality rates decreased because of the eradication and control of infectious diseases, due to such public health measures as provision of safe water and milk supplies and effective sewage disposal. With improved socioeconomic conditions, there came improved personal hygiene, housing, and nutrition. The care of health came to be seen in a wider context, embracing behavioral and environmental factors.

In contemporary society, we see an increasing interest in personal behavior, lifestyle, and the social and natural environment. The study and regulation of these are now recognized as indispensable elements in modern health care. In other words, health care can no longer be confined within the limits of the clinical model. Contemporary civilization can no longer ignore the impact of its technology on the conditions of life. Throughout modern history there has been a growing protest and challenge against the injury and degradation of the quality of life that has sometimes been the price we have paid for technological progress and efficiency. Through much of the past, this protest has been a demand for economic reform. But new ideals of humanity and society have thrown new light on these problems. Reform has come to aim not merely at escape from economic privation; it has become a striving for those conditions in which the best qualities of life may be attainable. To see this well-being as not merely incidental and peripheral to a humane society but as the indispensable element of modern health care is to adopt the eudaimonistic model of health.

The foregoing analysis of the four models of health has indicated the very great difference between the clinical model and the eudaimonistic model. The former is almost completely unrelated to anything beyond the structure and function of the organism, while the latter—in addition to these organic aspects—views people in the context of their complex social, environmental, and cultural relations. Adopting one or the other of these models of health care may have a significant bearing on the role of the nurse. The vastly expanded area of health care under the eudaimonistic model involves responsibilities in public health, primary care, health education, and research, all of which are included in the educational preparation of the nurse.

Conceiving health on the adaptive or eudaimonistic models means a vast expansion in the area of health care—an expansion into regions that are not traditionally regarded as the concern of the health professions, although increasing attention has been given to them in recent decades. For example, concern for the development and preservation of a congenial salutary environment is implicit in the adaptive model. Similarly, certain aspects of individual life have come to be seen as factors in health. Among these may be included stress on the job, the failures and frustrations of life, and alienation from social strata that provide opportunities for rewarding careers. In other words, under the eudaimonistic model all such failures in achievement and self-fulfillment are seen as assaults on health. Thus, the availability of opportunities for growth in education, vocation, and emotional maturity is viewed in this model as the concern of the health professions. This amounts to saying that these two models make the quality of life the major concern of the health professions.

Major Concerns of Professional Nurses
Under the Adaptive and Eudaimonistic Models

Such broad concerns lead to involvements in fundamental social and political policies that influence the role of nursing. These two models focus respectively on the natural and the social environments. As regards the natural environment, these models imply intervention of government in some form to:

1.   Ensure regulation, modification, and preservation of the physical environment.
2.   Institute social measures providing individuals with the knowledge and means for coping with adverse physical conditions.
3.   Undertake general public health education through school curricula and continuing adult education.

As regards the social environment, government would:

1.   Aim at the adoption of policies for expansion of opportunities in vocation, liberal education, and leisure time activities.
2.   Ensure suitable economic provisions for pursuing such educational and vocational advancements.
3.   Support institutions of continuing education such as colleges, museums, and libraries.
4.   Cultivate the general availability and use of physical fitness facilities.

In addition to the nursing skills required under the clinical model, the nurse's training generally embraces the broader concerns and skills of public health, psychological aspects, and general sociology of health care. These elements of training and education uniquely qualify the nurse as an effective agent in the functioning of these policies. Under the adaptive and eudaimonistic models, there will evidently result a variety of extensions and modifications of the nurse's role. One cannot anticipate all these at present, but among those that are clearly indicated will be intensified activities in the following areas:

1. *Health educator in schools and community centers.* Under conditions of modern civilization, most people require assistance and guidance in their personal health care. Of course, this need for instruc-

tion is especially acute in childhood. It has been said that what an individual does with his body from early childhood on has more influence over his health than anything nurses or physicians can do for him once he is ill.[5] The patterns of adult life related to obesity, dental caries, and iron-deficiency anemia are shaped in early childhood. Consequently, health education in childhood becomes a significant factor in community health.

Numerous other aspects of modern life play a determining role in the health of the individual. Most of these lie outside the purview of the clinical model with its emphasis on curative medicine. Nevertheless, adequate health care must include pervasive education and regulation with regard to these patterns of life in contemporary society. Alcohol and drug abuse, cigarette smoking, the unsafe and reckless use of automobiles, sedentary lifestyles, family disharmony, deficient diets—the list seems endless—these are among the characteristics of individual life within the scope of individual personal choice. Making that choice intelligent and informed becomes a paramount responsibility of health care—a responsibility that curative medicine, practiced within the context of the clinical model, is neither equipped nor able to bear. This health care opens a wider vista and engages a different type of nursing concern than is entailed in the clinical model. Thus, the enlarged scope of health care presents an enlarged role of practice for the nurse.

2. *Health officer with responsibilities for the detection of adverse environmental conditions in the community.* The nurse as health officer in the community would be responsible for evaluating the state of that community. Evaluations of the adequacy of recreational facilities and transportation systems are necessary in order to help ensure the quality of life in that community. Having inadequate transportation systems in an urban area leads to various hardships in family life. For example, parents may have to rise very early in the morning to get to their jobs on time, thereby leaving young children at home to prepare themselves for school: washing, dressing, preparing meals. Without specific supervision,·young children do not eat or dress properly. While these facts of daily life among the deprived and impoverished may appear trivial, nevertheless they are decisive factors in the high incidence of disease and a general deterioration of life manifested in such signs as retarded learning in school, apathy on the playground, and inability to concentrate. Thus, the kinds of community health problems identified by the nurse would go far

beyond the usual problems, such as common childhood diseases and venereal diseases.

3. *Diagnostic observer, teacher, and counselor of people in the community.* People seek out health practitioners not only when they are sick, but because they have difficulty coping with problems of life. In such cases, expertise in the problems of abnormal physiology is not enough. The practitioner interested in health has to cultivate skills in counseling and teaching in order to assist people in exploring the alternatives available to them and acting on the one most appropriate for their situation.

Within the context of the eudaimonistic model of health, the nursing interest would not be limited to the mere preservation of health within existing conditions, such as in providing essential medical services to the poor, but would strive to help provide opportunities for self-development, schooling, and so forth. Escape from frustration would be a part of health care. The nurse's task would be undertaken as part of a pervasive concern for the general well-being of people in happy, fulfilling patterns of life.

Unanswered Questions Concerning
the Expanded Role of Nurses

A sharper delineation of the so-called expanded role as distinguished from the traditional role of the nurse becomes possible when viewed within the context of the adaptive and eudaimonistic models of health. The subject of this expanded role for nurses has received much attention in other contexts (as in independent practice), but the literature on this topic has left certain vital questions unanswered.[6] It is not clear how these advocates of the expanded role relate the proposed change in scope of activity to the education of the nurse. Does the expanded role consist of the expanded use of knowledge and skills already possessed by the traditional nurse? Or does the expanded role entail a new and enlarged education and training in new skills that heretofore were not considered part of the traditional education and training of the nurse? Furthermore, similar questions arise concerning the specific functions entailed in the expanded role. Will the nurse perform functions traditionally restricted to the practice of the physician? Or does the nurse in this expanded role perform functions that are new and different from both those of the traditional nurse and those of the traditional physician? Is there, in other words, a new area of health care in which the new nursing practitioner will perform a distinctive role? The full meaning of an expanded role for nurses will not be clear until these questions are answered.

Whatever answers are reached, it is clear that curative nursing does not exhaust the role of the nurse. An important area of nursing is focused on the prevention of illness and the preservation of health. Such are the responsibilities of the nurses engaged in community health. With the evolution of public health, we have seen the emergence of the community health nurse with specialized knowledge in such fields as epidemiology, biostatistics, the social and behavioral sciences, which is applied in practice without infringing on the role of the physician. In the pursuit of programs of disease prevention and health education, the community health nurse exercises more or less autonomous decisions within the framework of the role as nurse. From this viewpoint, the community health nurse is already a professional, free of the supervision of the physician.

Such a new area of health care has been suggested in light of the adaptive and eudaimonistic models of health. The functions of the contemporary community health nurse need to be expanded into the areas suggested by these models, and more nurses would be needed for these tasks. In 1980, only 83,000 of 1.3 million nurses were practicing in public health.[7] The nurse with the expanded scope of practice in health care would be utilized most in those areas where the physician is absent. This new type of nurse is clearly distinct from the hospital and office nurses who practice for the most part under the control of physicians.

The assumption of these responsibilities means a corresponding change in education. The nurse has to be taught to stop thinking only clinically and to start thinking in terms of the adaptive and eudaimonistic models. The nurse would be steeped in the social philosophy underlying these two models. The nurse as key figure in the delivery of health care under this new education would become the guardian of the quality of life in the community.

Directions for Nursing Research

A number of facets of the idea of health awaiting further study are implicit in the foregoing inquiry. These are within the realm of nursing research and include:

1. The idea of optimal structure and optimal functioning of the human organism—what would be considered the "healthy"

anatomy and physiology of the organism. It is possible to outline the desirable anatomical and physiologic traits that are within the reach of most people. This would be considered the healthy physical state.

2.   The idea of the healthy environment with which the organism interacts. The environment would be of such a nature that the individual would be free of fear and terror. This implies a presence of social justice, economic security, and a favorable physical environment.

3.   The idea of the optimal outlook of the self on the self. The individual would have a favorable self-concept; he would be confident and disciplined; he would cultivate moral concepts like fairness, honesty, and love; he would have the capacity for sustained effort; he would have the courage to face risks of disappointment and physical injury; and he would have the courage to hold his convictions alone in the face of strong criticism. In short, individuals would develop a meaningful conception of life by which they would pursue their lives.

Ethical and Social Orientations

A comparative survey of the foregoing models suggests certain values related to individual and social action. Some ethical and social ideals may be seen as indicated by these values. The following paragraphs present in summary form the relative merits of these models with respect to (1) the scope of the underlying image of man, (2) the range of nursing responsibility entailed in these models, (3) the social perspectives implicit in them, and (4) the orientation of these models regarding the overall quality of life.

The four models of health can be viewed as four ways of looking at human life. As was stated earlier, these four ways can be seen as serial, or progressive, leading from the simplest to the most comprehensive outlook on man. This leads to corresponding four types of social policy with regard to health—each model of health providing the keynote or basis for social measures concerning the health of the community or nation. These policies entail decisions concerning a variety of administrative measures and institutions, including "environmental health (epidemic disease control, sanitary hygiene) and personal health (preventive medicine, social hygiene, social medicine, social insurance)."[8] The range and effectiveness of the foregoing measures depend to a great extent on the attitude and participation of the public in whose interest they are undertaken. Consequently, health education becomes a paramount factor in any public health policy.

The four models of health can be seen as defining the scope of interest and responsibility concerning health assumed by the community or government. The successive models of health—the clinical, the role-performance, the adaptive, the eudaimonistic—indicate four levels of public health.

Level I: Clinical Model.   The first level of public health sees its responsibility as limited to facilitating access to medical and nursing services in private offices, clinics, and the hospital in providing certain minimal protection from epidemics and other public risks of disease, such as unsanitary water supplies.

Level II: Role-Performance Model.   This includes the first level but goes beyond it for an interest in all those conditions that ensure the continued effective functioning of people in the community in their varied economic and social roles.

Level III: Adaptive Model.   This goes beyond the foregoing to provide the physical and cultural development and social insights that can prepare people for changes in the economic and social environment.

Level IV: Eudaimonistic Model.   At this level, the community assumes the responsibility for the foregoing, but in addition it aims to provide individuals with the physical and social conditions and the quality of life in which they can achieve the fullest realization and expression of their potentialities.

It becomes evident that education must play an increasing role in these successive levels. In many ways, a healthy lifestyle is a program of self-help. That is, it is dependent on individual responsibility. Most nurses and physicians focus on patients after they have already suffered physiologic damage. Considering the conditions most often causing death in the population today—heart disease, cancer, stroke—physicians and nurses often offer only a band-aid approach. They rarely deal with the fundamental causes of poor health, such as inadequate diet, stress, or personal habits such as smoking. Several investigations have stressed the extent to which health is influenced by individual lifestyle and behavior. In 1972, Belloc and Breslow published a study of 7,000 California adults that showed that good health is related to certain specified personal habits. These habits appear to preserve good health despite the impact of increasing age. The study showed that the physical health of the individuals who followed all the recommended practices was about the same as that of very much younger persons.[9]

This study emphasizes that some of the fundamental reasons for poor health lie within the realm of individual personal responsibility. Therefore, an important aim of social policy lies in the area of health education: cultivating attitudes of self-care, and imparting the appropriate knowledge dealing with health maintenance, health promotion, and prevention of disease. Such a policy can provide the basis for a higher quality of life.

In light of the eudaimonistic model, public health policy must go beyond health education. It must concern itself with the design and provision of healthy social and physical surroundings. Thus, social policy proceeds from the conception of the healthy individual to the idea of a "healthy" society—a society that can provide the conditions and services required for the fullest growth and fulfillment of its members.

Insofar as Maslow's idea of the self-actualizing person is central to this model, an important qualification should be added. This concept of self-actualization may be understood to mean that the self-actualizing person is antecedently fixed and complete in all the potentialities and that a "healthy" life consists in the unfolding or realization of these potential traits. Such interpretation ignores the fact that the "self," the "character" of a person, is capable of change; that, in fact, it does change under the impact of experience. In other words, one must invoke the adaptive model to stress that growth is not only the actualization of what was antecedently present as potentiality, but that growth also entails genuine novelty. New qualities of self and personality emerge through experience and intelligent self-discipline.

Conclusion

The foregoing discussion of implications of the models of health has not treated the four models with equal attention. The reason for this lies in the differing significance of the four models in relation to the prospects for change in current health care. The clinical model and the role-performance model are, in fact, exemplified in current and traditional practice. The medical profession has been implicitly guided by the clinical model of health for many centuries. The attitude of large numbers of laymen, as well as the aim of medical and nursing therapy in an occupational health context, is conceived on the patterns of the role-performance model. In the conception and presentation of the adaptive and eudaimonistic models, proposals for innovation were being implicitly formulated. The works of Dubos and Maslow with regard to health care are still in the nature of innovations, perhaps of revolutions, in nursing practice. Therefore, this discussion of implications has focused on the adaptive and eudaimonistic models. It is their implications that carry a certain urgency because they are, in fact, anticipations of changes in practice that would result from a widespread adoption of these two models as directives of health care.

Notes

Bibliography

Index

NOTES

Chapter 1. Introduction

1. Cf. Brockington in the *Encyclopaedia Britannica*, 1968 ed., s.v. "Public Health," states that historically the phrase *public health* has been used to encompass both environmental health (epidemic disease control, sanitary hygiene) and personal health (preventive medicine, social hygiene, social medicine, social insurance). Within the past few years, the phrase *community health* has been used to encompass similar areas. In this work, these phrases are used interchangeably.
2. Used in this sense, health is a relative concept. States of health are measured against some standard or ideal of health. The models of health discussed in this book are standards of health.
3. Gradation is a generic concept. Any sequence of things arranged in the order of some appraised quality is a gradation. Some gradations are continuous, that is, an unbroken sequence of things arranged so that between any two points there is always an intermediate point. But some gradations are discrete, that is, discontinuous as when we arrange people in order of grade in the army. There are no ranks (no intermediate points) between captain and major, etc. Thus, the idea of gradation embraces the notions of discrete and continuous. Sometimes the concept gradation will be used in its most general form. At other times, the term continuum will be used to mean an unbroken series.
4. The word *comparative* is used in the strict technical sense. Carl G. Hempel, *Fundamentals of Concept Formation*, p. 54, states, "a comparative concept allows for a 'more or less': it provides for a gradual transition from cases where the characteristic is nearly or entirely absent to others where it is very marked."
5. *Encyclopaedia Britannica*, 1956 ed., s.v. "Medicine."
6. Marc Lalonde, *A New Perspective on the Health of Canadians*, p. 15.
7. U.S., Department of Health, Education, and Welfare, *Forward Plan for Health*, p. 117.
8. George Rosen, *From Medical Police to Social Medicine*, pp. 64–67.

9. Ibid., p. 27, and Shryock, *Nursing*, pp. 35–36.
10. W.H.S. Jones, trans., "Decorum," in *Hippocrates*, vol. 2, p. 299.

Chapter 2. Nursing and Medicine

1. See, for example, S.G. Blaxland Stubbs and E.W. Bligh, *Sixty Centuries of Health and Physick*; Theodor Puschmann, *A History of Medical Education*; Anne L. Austin, *History of Nursing Source Book*; and Richard H. Shryock, *The History of Nursing*.
2. Authorities date the Charaka Samhita anywhere from 500 B.C. to 200 A.D. Most appear to place it in the first century A.D.
3. Written records of ancient Babylonia appear only on clay tablets with language symbols engraved on them.
4. Arturo Castigione, *A History of Medicine*, p. 40.
5. Stubbs and Bligh, *Sixty Centuries*, pp. 12–13.
6. Nandkumar H. Keswani, "Medical Education in India Since Ancient Times," p. 333.
7. Puschmann, *History*, p. 13.
8. Austin, *Source Book*, p. 26.
9. Ibid., p. 27, and Shryock, *Nursing*, pp. 35–36.
10. W.H.S. Jones, trans., "Decorum," in *Hippocrates*, vol. 2, p. 299.
11. Puschmann, *History*, p. 61.
12. Will Durant, *Caesar and Christ*, pp. 627–28.
13. G.G. Coulton, *The Medieval Scene*, p. 8.
14. Ibid., p. 7.
15. Puschmann, *History*, pp. 145–46.
16. Shryock, *Nursing*, p. 96.
17. For a more complete analysis of care in the nineteenth century, see Dorothy A. Sheahan, "The Social Origins of American Nursing and Its Movement into the University: A Microcosmic Approch," pp. 25–100.
18. D. Diderot and J. d'Alembert, *Le Rond D'Encyclopédie*, s.v. "Infirmier," p. 707.
19. Shryock, *Nursing*, p. 232.
20. See for example, M. Adelaide Nutting and Lavinia L. Dock, *A History of Nursing*, vol. 2, pp. 62–100.
21. Philip A. Kalisch and Beatrice J. Kalisch, *The Advance of American Nursing*, pp. 28–30; Lois A. Monteiro, ed., *Letters of Florence Nightingale*, p. 23; Nutting and Dock, *History*, vol. 1, pp. 499–524; Abby H. Woolsey, *A Century of Nursing*, pp. 3–133.
22. Kalisch and Kalisch, *Advance*, p. 161; Monteiro, *Letters*, p. 29.
23. Florence Nightingale, *Notes on Nursing: What It Is and What It Is Not*, passim; Nutting and Dock, *History*, vol. 2, pp. 172–206.
24. "Report of the Committee on the Training of Nurses," p. 161.
25. Kalisch and Kalisch, *Advance*, p. 87.

Chapter 3. Health as Paideia

1. B. Jowett, trans. *The Dialogues of Plato*, 1:156c. 1–36.
2. Ibid., 3:270c. 107–90.
3. Werner Jaeger, *Paideia: The Ideals of Greek Culture*, vol. 1, p. 306.
4. William Arthur Heidel, *Hippocratic Medicine: Its Spirit and Method*, p. 34.
5. Francis Adams, trans., *The Genuine Works of Hippocrates*, pp. 19–41.
6. Ludwig Edelstein, *Ancient Medicine: Selected Papers*, p. 315.
7. Jaeger, *Paideia*, vol. 1, p. 307.
8. Philip Wheelwright, ed., *The PreSocratics*, pp. 1–40.
9. Ibid., pp. 41–42.
10. Jaeger, *Paideia*, vol. 1, p. 306.
11. Ibid., vol. 3, p. 22
12. Ibid., p. 27.
13. Edelstein, *Ancient Medicine*, pp. 303–16.
14. Crane Brinton, *Ideas and Men*, 2nd ed., p. 289.
15. Ibid., 1st ed., p. 380.
16. Ibid., pp. 385–86.
17. Ibid., p. 386.
18. Jeremy Bentham, *The Principles of Morals and Legislation*, p. 1.
19. Ibid., p. 3.
20. *The Times*, 8 July 1854, quoted in S.E. Finer, *The Life and Times of Sir Edwin Chadwick*, pp. 1–2.
21. George Rosen, *A History of Public Health*, pp. 293, 332.

Chapter 5. Clinical Model

1. F.C. Redlich, "Editorial Reflections on the Concepts of Health and Disease," p. 270.
2. W.R. Barclay, "Hypertension: A Major Medical Care Challenge," p. 2327.
3. The term *homeostasis* was coined by W.B. Cannon, who extended the work of Claude Bernard.
4. Claude Bernard, *Phenomena 1876*, quoted in J.M.D. Olmsted and E. Harris Olmsted, *Claude Bernard & The Experimental Method in Medicine*, pp. 107–08, 224–25.
5. Olmsted and Olmsted, *Claude Bernard*, p. 224.
6. Norbert Wiener, "The Concept of Homeostasis in Medicine," p. 154.
7. Stephen Toulmin, "Concepts of Function and Mechanism in Medicine and Medical Science," p. 59.
8. C. Daly King, "The Meaning of Normal," p. 494.
9. Stephen Toulmin, "On the Nature of the Physicians' Understanding," p. 40.

10. Ibid., p. 47.
11. Ibid., p. 43.
12. Samuel Gorovitz and Alasdair MacIntyre, "Toward a Theory of Medical Fallibility," pp. 64–65.
13. Alvan R. Feinstein, *Clinical Judgment*, p. 24.

Chapter 6. Role-Performance Model

1. Talcott Parsons, "Definitions of Health and Illness in the Light of American Values and Social Structure," p. 107.
2. Andrew C. Twaddle, "The Concept of Health Status," p. 31.
3. Robert N. Wilson, *The Sociology of Health*, p. 6.
4. David Mechanic, *Medical Sociology*, p. 57.
5. Twaddle, "Health Status," p. 31.
6. Parsons, "Health and Illness," p. 107.
7. Mechanic, *Medical Sociology*, p. 78.
8. Lena DiCicco and Dorrian Apple, "Health Needs and Opinions of Older Adults," pp. 26–39.
9. Earl Lomon Koos, *The Health of Regionville*, p. 35.
10. Edward A. Suchman, "Stages of Illness and Medical Care," p. 118.
11. Michael Grossman, "The Correlation Between Health and Schooling," pp. 166–68.
12. Robert Nisbet, *The Social Bond*, p. 148.
13. William Goode, "A Theory of Role Strain," p. 18.
14. *International Encyclopedia of the Social Sciences*, 1968 ed., s.v. "Role: Psychological Aspects."
15. Nisbet, *The Social Bond*, p. 152.
16. Goode, "Role Strain," p. 10.
17. Parsons, "Health and Illness," p. 117.

Chapter 7. Adaptive Model

1. René Dubos, *Mirage of Health*, passim; *Man Adapting*, pp. 1–109, 163–456; *A God Within*, pp. 234–55. *Mirage of Health*, volume 22 in *World Perspectives*, planned and edited by Ruth Nanda Anshen. Copyright © 1959 by René Dubos. Reprinted by permission of Harper & Row, Publishers, Inc.
2. Dubos, *Mirage*, p. 33.
3. Ibid., p. 39.
4. Ibid., pp. 39–40.
5. John Dewey, *Democracy and Education*, p. 56.
6. A detailed discussion of this social theory is presented in Richard Hofstadter, *Social Darwinism in American Thought*.

7. Dewey, *Democracy*, p. 56.
8. Dubos. *Mirage*, p. 2.
9. Dubos, *A God Within*, p. 244.
10. Dubos, *Mirage*, p. 22.
11. Ibid., p. 231.
12. Dewey, *Democracy*, p. 49.
13. Ibid., p. 206.
14. Dubos, *Mirage*, pp. 89–90.
15. Ibid., p. 136.
16. W.H.S. Jones, trans., *Hippocrates*, vol. 1, p. ix.
17. Dubos, *A God Within*, p. 181.
18. Daphne A. Roe, *A Plague of Corn: The Social History of Pellagra*, p. 132.
19. For a detailed presentation of this topic, see Norbert Wiener, *Cybernetics*; W. Ross Ashby, *Design for a Brain: The Origin of Adaptive Behavior*.
20. *Webster's Dictionary*, 1934, s.v. "thermostat."
21. John A. Ryle, quoted in Iago Galdston, *The Meaning of Social Medicine*, p. 14.
22. This does not mean that health is a *subjective* concept. Dubos takes great care to show that there is a rational basis for health in that everyone needs certain physical and environmental conditions in order to be healthy.

Chapter 8. Eudaimonistic Model

1. Abraham H. Maslow, "Health as Transcendence of Environment," pp. 1–7; *Toward a Psychology of Being*, passim; *Motivation and Personality*, pp. 19–104, 149–202, 265–80; and *The Farther Reaches of Human Nature*, pp. 3–53. *Motivation and Personality*, second edition, copyright © 1970 by Abraham Maslow. Reprinted by permission of Harper & Row, Publishers, Inc.
2. J.H. Woodger, *Biological Principles: A Critical Study*, pp. 259–72. Reprinted by permission of Humanities Press, Inc.
3. Ludwig von Bertalanffy, *Modern Theories of Development: An Introduction to Theoretical Biology*, p. 72.
4. de Beer, *Growth*, p. 112, quoted in Woodger, *Biological Principles*, p. 258.
5. René Descartes, *Discourse on Method, Optics, Geometry, and Meteorology*, pp. 16–17.
6. Kurt Goldstein, *The Organism: A Holistic Approach to Biology Derived from Pathological Data in Man*, p. 68.
7. John Herman Randall, Jr., *The Making of the Modern Mind*, p. 482.
8. John Herman Randall, Jr., and Justus Buchler, *Philosophy: An Introduction*, p. 202.
9. Jacques Loeb, *The Mechanistic Conception of Life*, p. 31.

10. Ibid., p. 62.
11. William McDougall, *The Riddle of Life: A Survey of Theories*, p. 149.
12. Giovanni Blandino, *Theories on the Nature of Life*, p. 161.
13. Bertalanffy, *Modern Theories*, p. 46.
14. Ibid., p. 8.
15. Ibid., p. 65.
16. Goldstein, *A Holistic Approach*, p. 121.
17. Ibid., p. 46.
18. Ibid., p. 57.
19. Ibid., p. 214.
20. Ibid., p. vii.
21. McDougall, *The Riddle of Life*, p. 174.
22. Francis Crick, *Of Molecules and Men*, p. 13.
23. M. Brewster Smith, "On Self-Actualization: A Transambivalent Examination of a Focal Theme in Maslow's Psychology," pp. 17–33.
24. Ibid., p. 24.
25. Edward L. Koos, *The Health of Regionville*, pp. 30–52.
26. Leo Strole et al., *Mental Health in the Metropolis: The Midtown Manhattan Study*, p. 151.
27. Lena DiCicco and Dorrian Apple, "Health Needs and Opinions of Older Adults," pp. 26–39.
28. *Encyclopedia of Philosophy*, 1972 ed., s.v. "American Philosophy."
29. Smith, "On Self-Actualization," p. 25.
30. These views are developed in John Dewey, *Reconstruction in Philosophy*, p. 184, and *Democracy and Education*, p. 49.

Chapter 9. Structure and Interrelationships of the Four Models

1. Institute of Medicine, *Nursing and Nursing Education*, p. 27.
2. Rick J. Carlson, *The End of Medicine*, passim; Kerr L. White, "Health Problems and Priorities and the Health Professions," pp. 560–66; Rick J. Carlson and Robert Cunningham, eds., *Future Directions in Health Care: A New Public Policy*, pp. xiii–xviii; and Thomas McKeown, "Behavioral and Environmental Determinants of Health and Their Implications for Public Policy," pp. 21–37.
3. Carlson and Cunningham, *Future Directions*, p. xv.
4. See, for example, American Nurses' Association and the American Academy of Pediatrics, "Guidelines for Short-Term Continuing Education Programs for Pediatric Nurse Associates," pp. 509–12; A. Elizabeth Walker, "PRIMEX—The Family Nurse Practitioner Program," pp. 176–83 [listed in Table of Contents as beginning on p. 207]; Anita O'Toole, "The Expanded Role: Issues and Opportunities for Nursing" (paper presented at the biennial convention of the American Nurses' Association, Honolulu, Hawaii, June 1978).

5. Earl Ubell, "Health Behavior Change: A Political Model," p. 210.
6. M. Lucille Kinlein, "Independent Nurse Practitioner," pp. 22–24; Ada K. Jacox and Catherine M. Norris, eds., *Organizing for Independent Nursing Practice*, p. 225.
7. Institute of Medicine, *Nursing and Nursing Education*, p. 58.
8. *Encyclopaedia Britannica*, 1968 ed., s.v. "Public Health."
9. Nedra B. Belloc and Lester Breslow, "Relationship of Physical Health Status and Health Practices," pp. 409–21.

BIBLIOGRAPHY

Adams, Francis, trans. *The Genuine Works of Hippocrates*. Baltimore: Williams & Wilkins Co., 1939.

American Nurses' Association and the American Academy of Pediatrics. "Guidelines for Short-Term Continuing Education Programs for Pediatric Nurse Associates." *American Journal of Nursing* 71 (1971): 509–12.

Ashby, W. Ross. *Design for a Brain: The Origin of Adaptive Behavior*. 2nd ed. rev. New York: John Wiley and Sons, 1960.

Austin, Anne L. *History of Nursing Source Book*. New York: G.P. Putnam's Sons, 1957.

Barclay, W.R. "Hypertension: A Major Medical Care Challenge." *Journal of the American Medical Association* 235 (1976): 2327.

Beckner, Morton. *The Biological Way of Thought*. New York: Columbia University Press, 1959.

Belloc, Nedra B. and Breslow, Lester. "Relationship of Physical Health Status and Health Practices." *Preventive Medicine* 1 (1972): 409–21.

Bentham, Jeremy. *The Principles of Morals and Legislation*. New York: Hafner Publishing Co., 1948.

Bertalanffy, Ludwig von. *Problems of Life*. London: Watts & Co., 1952.

———. *Modern Theories of Development: An Introduction to Theoretical Biology*. Translated by J.H. Woodger. New York: Harper & Bros., 1962.

Blandino, Giovanni. *Theories on the Nature of Life*. New York: Philosophical Library, 1969.

Brinton, Crane. *Ideas and Men: The Story of Western Thought*. New York: Prentice-Hall, 1st ed., 1950; 2nd ed. 1963.

Burnet, John. *Early Greek Philosophy*. London: Adam and Charles Black, 1892.

Carlson, Rick J. *The End of Medicine*. New York: John Wiley and Sons, 1975.

Carlson, Rick J. and Cunningham, Robert, eds. *Future Directions in Health Care: A New Public Policy*. Cambridge, Mass.: Ballinger Publishing Company, 1978.

Castigione, Arturo. *A History of Medicine*. New York: Alfred A. Knopf, 1958.

Chadwick, Edwin. *Report on the Sanitary Condition of the Labouring Popula-*

tion of Great Britain. Edited and with an introduction by M.W. Flinn. Edinburgh: Edinburgh University Press, 1965.

Coulton, G.G. *The Medieval Scene.* Cambridge: The University Press, 1930.

———. *Medieval Panorama.* New York: Macmillian, 1938.

Crick, Francis. *Of Molecules and Men.* Seattle: University of Washington Press, 1966.

Descartes, René. *Discourse on Method, Optics, Geometry, and Meteorology.* Translated by Paul J. Olscamp. Indianapolis: Bobbs-Merrill, 1965.

Dewey, John. *Democracy and Education.* New York: Macmillan, 1916.

———. *Reconstruction in Philosophy.* Enl. ed. Boston: Beacon Press, 1948.

Dewey, John and Tufts, James H. *Ethics.* New York: Henry Holt and Co., 1908.

DiCicco, Lena and Apple, Dorrian. "Health Needs and Opinions of Older Adults." In *Sociological Studies of Health and Illness,* edited by Dorrian Apple, pp. 26–39. New York: McGraw-Hill, 1960.

Diderot, D. and d'Alembert, J. *Le Rond D'. Encyclopédie.* New Haven, Conn.: Research Publications Inc., Film 2371, Reel 990, No. 10827, v. 8, 1751–65, s.v. "Infirmier," pp. 707–08.

Dubos, René. *Mirage of Health: Utopias, Progress & Biological Change.* Vol. 22 in *World Perspectives,* planned and edited by Ruth Nanda Anshen. 1959. New York: Harper & Row, reprint ed., 1979.

———. *Man Adapting.* New Haven, Conn.: Yale University Press, 1965.

———. *A God Within.* New York: Charles Scribner's Sons, 1972.

Durant, Will. *The Life of Greece.* New York: Simon and Schuster, 1939.

———. *The Age of Faith.* New York: Simon and Schuster, 1950.

———. *Caesar and Christ.* New York: Simon and Schuster, 1944.

Edelstein, Ludwig. *Ancient Medicine:-Selected Papers.* Edited by Oswei Temkin and C. Lillian Temkin. Translated by C. Lillian Temkin. Baltimore: Johns Hopkins University Press, 1967.

Encyclopaedia Britannica. 1956 ed., s.v. "Medicine."

Encyclopaedia Britannica. 1968 ed., s.v. "Public Health."

Encyclopedia of Philosophy. 1972 ed., s.v. "American Philosophy."

Encyclopedia of Philosophy. 1967 ed., s.v. "Baron d'Holbach, Paul-Henri Thiry."

Engelhardt, H.T., Jr. "The Concept of Health and Disease." In *Evaluation and Explanation in the Biomedical Sciences,* edited by H.T. Engelhardt and S.F. Spicker, pp. 125–41. Dordrecht-Holland: D. Reidel Publishing Co., 1975.

Feinstein, Alvan R. *Clinical Judgment.* Huntington, N.Y.: Robert E. Krieger, 1967.

Finer, S.E. *The Life and Times of Sir Edwin Chadwick.* 2nd ed. New York: Barnes & Noble, 1970.

Galdston, Iago, ed. *Social Medicine: Its Derivations and Objectives.* New York: Commonwealth Fund, 1949.

———. *The Meaning of Social Medicine.* Cambridge, Mass.: Harvard University Press, 1954.

Goldstein, Kurt. *The Organism: A Holistic Approach to Biology Derived from Pathological Data in Man.* Boston: Beacon Press, 1963.

Goode, William. "A Theory of Role Strain." In *The Dynamics of Modern Society*, edited by William Goode, pp. 7–22. New York: Atherton Press, 1966.

Gorovitz, Samuel and MacIntyre, Alasdair. "Toward a Theory of Medical Fallibility." *Journal of Medicine and Philosophy* 1 (1976): 51–71.

Grossman, Michael. "The Correlation Between Health and Schooling." In *Household Production and Consumption*, edited by Nestor E. Terleckyi, pp. 147–211. New York: National Bureau of Economic Research, 1975.

Heidel, William. *Hippocratic Medicine: Its Spirit and Method*. New York: Columbia University Press, 1941.

Hempel, Carl G. *Fundamentals of Concept Formation*. Chicago: University of Chicago Press, 1952.

Hofstadter, Richard. *Social Darwinism in American Thought*. Rev. ed. New York: George Braziller, 1959.

Institute of Medicine. *Nursing and Nursing Education: Public Policies and Private Actions*. Washington, D.C.: National Academy Press, 1983.

Jacox, Ada K. and Norris, Catherine M., eds. *Organizing for Independent Nursing Practice*. New York: Appleton-Century-Crofts, 1977.

Jaeger, Werner. *Paideia: The Ideals of Greek Culture*. 2nd ed. Translated by Gilbert Highet. Vol. 1: *Archaic Greece: The Mind of Athens*, Vol. 3: *The Conflict of Cultural Ideals in the Age of Plato*. New York: Oxford University Press, 1945.

————. *The Theology of the Early Greek Philosophers*. The Gifford Lectures, 1936. Oxford: Clarendon Press, 1948.

Jones, W.H.S., trans. *Hippocrates*. The Loeb Classical Library. Vols. 1, 2. London: William Heinemann, 1923.

Jowett, B., trans. *The Dialogues of Plato*. 4th ed. Oxford: Clarendon Press, 1953.

Kalisch, Philip A. and Kalisch, Beatrice J. *The Advance of American Nursing*. Boston: Little, Brown and Co., 1978.

Keswani, Nandkumar H. "Medical Education in Ancient India Since Ancient Times." In *The History of Medical Education*, edited by C.D. O'Malley, pp. 329–66. Berkeley: University of California Press, 1970.

King, C. Daly. "The Meaning of Normal." *Yale Journal of Biology and Medicine* 17 (1941–45): 493–501.

Kinlein, M. Lucille. "Independent Nurse Practitioner." *Nursing Outlook* 20 (1972): 22–24.

Koos, Earl L. *The Health of Regionville*. New York: Columbia University Press, 1954.

Lalonde, Marc. *A New Perspective on the Health of Canadians*. Ottawa: Ministry of National Health and Welfare, 1974.

La Mettrie, Julien Offray de. *L'Homme Machine*. Edited by Aram Vartanian. Princeton, N.J.: Princeton University Press, 1960.

Lewis, R.A. *Edwin Chadwick and the Public Health Movement: 1832–1854*. London: Longmans, Green & Co., 1952.

Loeb, Jacques. *The Mechanistic Conception of Life*. Chicago: University of Chicago Press, 1918.

McDougall, William. *Body and Mind*. 8th ed. London: Methuen & Co., 1938.

————. *The Riddle of Life: A Survey of Theories*. London: Methuen & Co., 1938.

McKeown, Thomas. "Behavioral and Environmental Determinants of Health and Their Implications for Public Policy." In *Future Directions in Health Care: A New Public Policy*, edited by Rick J. Carlson and Robert Cunningham, pp. 21–37. Cambridge, Mass.: Ballinger Publishing Co., 1978.

Maslow, Abraham H. "Health as Transcendence of Environment." *Journal of Humanistic Psychology* 1 (1961): 1–7.

————. *Toward a Psychology of Being*. Princeton, N.J.: Van Nostrand, 1962.

————. *Motivation and Personality*. 2nd ed. New York: Harper & Row, 1970.

————. *The Farther Reaches of Human Nature*. New York: Viking Press, 1971.

Mechanic, David. *Medical Sociology*. New York: Free Press, 1968.

Monteiro, Lois A., ed. *Letters of Florence Nightingale*. Boston: Boston University Nursing Archive, 1974.

Murphy, E.M. *The Logic of Medicine*. Baltimore: Johns Hopkins University Press, 1976.

Nightingale, Florence. *Notes on Nursing: What It Is and What It Is Not*. Facsimile reprint of 1860 ed. Phildelphia: University of Pennsylvania Printing Office, 1965.

Nisbet, Robert. *The Social Bond*. New York: Alfred A. Knopf, 1970.

Nutting, M. Adelaide and Dock, Lavinia L. *A History of Nursing: The Evolution of Nursing Systems from the Earliest Times to the Foundation of the First English and American Training Schools for Nurses*. 2 vols. New York: G.P. Putnam's Sons, 1935.

Olmsted, J.M.D. and Olmsted, E. Harris. *Claude Bernard & The Experimental Method in Medicine*. New York: Henry Schuman, 1952.

O'Toole, Anita. "The Expanded Role: Issues and Opportunities for Nursing." Paper presented at the biennial convention of the American Nurses' Association, Honolulu, Hawaii, June 1978.

Parsons, Talcott. "Definitions of Health and Illness in the Light of American Values and Social Structure." In *Patients, Physicians and Illness*, edited by E. Gartly Jaco, pp. 107–27. New York: Free Press, 1972.

Puschmann, Theodor. *A History of Medical Education*. Translated and edited by Evan H. Hare. New York: Hafner Publishing Co., 1966.

Randall, John H., Jr. *The Making of the Modern Mind*. Rev. ed. Boston: Houghton Mifflin, 1940.

Randall, John H., Jr. and Buchler, Justus. *Philosophy: An Introduction*. New York: Barnes & Noble, 1971.

Redlich, F.C. "Editorial Reflections on the Concepts of Health and Disease." *Journal of Medicine and Philosophy* 1 (1976): 269–80.

"Report of the Committee on the Training of Nurses." *Transactions of the American Medical Association*. 20 (1869): 161–74.

Richardson, Benjamin W. *The Health of Nations: A Review of the Works of Edwin Chadwick*. 2 vols. London: Dawsons of Pall Mall, 1965.

Roe, Daphne A. *A Plague of Corn: The Social History of Pellagra*. Ithaca: Cornell University Press, 1973.

Rosen, George. *A History of Public Health*. New York: MD Publications, 1958.
————. *From Medical Police to Social Medicine*. New York: Science History Publications, 1974.
Ryle, John A. "The Meaning of Normal." In *Concepts of Medicine*, edited by Brandon Lush, pp. 137–49. Oxford: Pergamon Press, 1961.
Sheahan, Dorothy A. "The Social Origins of American Nursing and Its Movement into the University: A Microcosmic Approach." Vol. 1–2. Doctoral dissertation, New York University, 1980.
Shorter Oxford English Dictionary of Historical Principles. 3rd ed. s.v. "Disease."
Shryock, Richard H. *The History of Nursing*. Philadelphia: W.B. Saunders Co., 1959.
Sigerist, Henry E. *A History of Medicine*. Vol. 2: *Early Greek, Hindu, and Persian Medicine*. New York: Oxford University Press, 1961.
Singer, Charles. *Greek Biology and Greek Medicine*. Oxford: Clarendon Press, 1922.
————. *A Short History of Medicine*. New York: Oxford University Press, 1928.
Smith, M. Brewster. "On Self-Actualization: A Transambivalent Examination of a Focal Theme in Maslow's Psychology." *Journal of Humanistic Psychology* 13 (1973): 17–33.
Strachey, Lytton. *Eminent Victorians*. New York: Knickerbocker Press, 1918, pp. 135–203.
Strole, Leo; Langner, Thomas S.; Michael, Stanley T.; Opler, Marvin K; and Rennie, Thomas A.C. *Mental Health in the Metropolis: The Midtown Manhattan Study*. New York: McGraw-Hill, 1962.
Stubbs, S.G. Blaxland and Bligh, E.W. *Sixty Centuries of Health and Physick*. New York: Paul B. Haeber, 1931.
Suchman, Edward A. "Stages of Illness and Medical Care." *Journal of Health and Human Behavior* 5–6 (1964–65): 114–28.
Taylor, Henry Osborn. *Greek Biology and Medicine*. New York: Cooper Square Publishers, 1963.
Toulmin, Stephen. "Concepts of Function and Mechanism in Medicine and Medical Science." In *Evaluation and Explanation in the Biomedical Sciences*, edited by H.T. Engelhardt and S.F. Spicker, pp. 51–66. Dordrecht-Holland: D. Reidel Publishing Co., 1975.
————. "On the Nature of the Physicians' Understanding." *Journal of Medicine and Philosophy* 1 (1976): 32–50.
Twaddle, Andrew C. "The Concept of Health Status." *Social Science and Medicine* 8 (1974): 29–38.
Ubell, Earl. "Health Behavior Change: A Political Model." *Preventive Medicine* 1 (1972): 209–21.
U.S., Department of Health, Education, and Welfare. *Forward Plan for Health*. Report prepared by the Public Health Service. Washington, D.C.: Government Printing Office, June 1975.
Walker, A. Elizabeth. "PRIMEX—The Family Nurse Practitioner Program." In *The Expanded Role of the Nurse*, edited by Mary H. Browning and Edith

P. Lewis, pp. 176–83. New York: American Journal of Nursing Co., 1973 [listed in Table of Contents as beginning on p. 207].

Webster's Unabridged Dictionary. 1934 ed., s.v. "Thermostat."

Wheelwright, Philip, ed. *The PreSocratics.* New York: Odyssey Press, 1966.

Wiener, Norbert. *Cybernetics.* New York: John Wiley and Sons, 1948.

————. "The Concept of Homeostasis in Medicine." *Concepts of Medicine,* edited by Brandon Lush, pp. 150–58. Oxford: Pergamon Press, 1961.

Wilson, Robert N. *The Sociology of Health.* New York: Random House, 1970.

Woodger, J.H. *Biological Principles: A Critical Study.* London: Routledge & Kegan Paul, 1929; reissue ed., Atlantic Highlands, N.J.: Humanities Press, 1967.

Woolsey, Abby H. *A Century of Nursing.* New York: G.P. Putnam's Sons, 1950.

INDEX

Goldberger, Joseph, 66
Goldstein, Kurt, 78–79
Governmental policy, 28–30
Gradation of health-illness, 2; definition of, 109n
Greek philosophy, 2, 23–26, 84
Gross, Samuel, 17
Grossman, Michael, 51
Growth, human, 63, 86–87, 90–91, 97
Guy's Hospital, London, 15

Haldane, J. B. S., 78
Hammurabi Code, 8
Happiness, 61, 100
Health, 22–30, 31–33, 34–35, 43–44, 48–53, 55–57, 61–64, 69, 72–74, 80–85, 87–88, 89–105; cycle, 18–19; education, 97–99, 103–04
Health-Illness Continuum, 31–32, 44, 47
Hempel, Carl G., 109n
Heredity, 35–36, 38
Hippocratic era, 10, 23–26, 30, 64, 65–66, 88
Hofstadter, Richard, 112n
Holism, 74–80
Homeostasis, 35–38, 91, 111n
Hospitals, 9, 12, 14–15, 92–93, 101
Housekeeping functions of nursing, 21
Human perfectability, 26–27

Institute of Nursing, London, 15
Intrusion of foreign substances, 35, 38–39
Iteration, 82

Jaeger, Werner, 2, 30
Jefferson, Thomas, 61

Koch, Robert, 64–65
Koos, Earl Lomon, 51, 83

Laboratory analysis, 41–42
Lalonde, Mark, 4
La Mettrie, Julien, 34–35
Locke, John, 26–27, 30
Love, 73, 82, 102

McDougall, William, 77–78, 80
Maslow, Abraham H., 32, 57, 72–74, 80–88, 105

May, Franz, 14–15
Mechanic, David, 49
Mechanistic conception of nature, 23, 34, 46–47, 74–80
Medicine as ways of restoring and preserving health, 3
Metchnikoff, Elie, 62
Model, 31–33; definition of, 2–3
Monasteries, 12–13

Naturalistic philosophy, 25–26, 30
New England Hospital for Women and Children, 17
Newton, Isaac, 26, 30
Nightingale, Florence, 16, 110n
Normal, concepts of, 39–43, 48–49, 54
Nurse liberation movement, 21
Nurse practitioners, 18–20, 21, 94–95
Nurse's profession, 3, 93–95, 100–01
Nursing: as an art, 16; history of, 7–21; practice, 5–6, 7–9, 33, 91–93; research, 101–02; school curricula, 92, 94

Oblates of Florence, 13
Occupational health, 32
Orderly, 95
Organismic biological doctrine, 78
Organization, in physiology, 37

Paideia, 22–30; definition of, 2
Parsons, Talcott, 32, 48–50, 55
Pasteur, Louis, 29, 64–65
Pathophysiology, 22–23, 40, 44, 47
Pellagra, 66–67
Pettenkofer, Max von, 62
Phenylketonuria, 38
Philosophical Radicals, 27–28
Physical fitness, 98
Physiology, 1, 3, 4, 40, 42, 102
Plato, 23, 25, 26, 72, 84–85, 88
Poor Clares, 13
Popularization of medical knowledge, 24
Potentiality, 85–87
Practical nurse, 95
Preventive medicine, 26, 30, 33, 102
Psychiatric clinical specialists, 19
Public health. *See* Community health
Puritanism, 84